The Mediterranean Diet Cookbook for Beginners

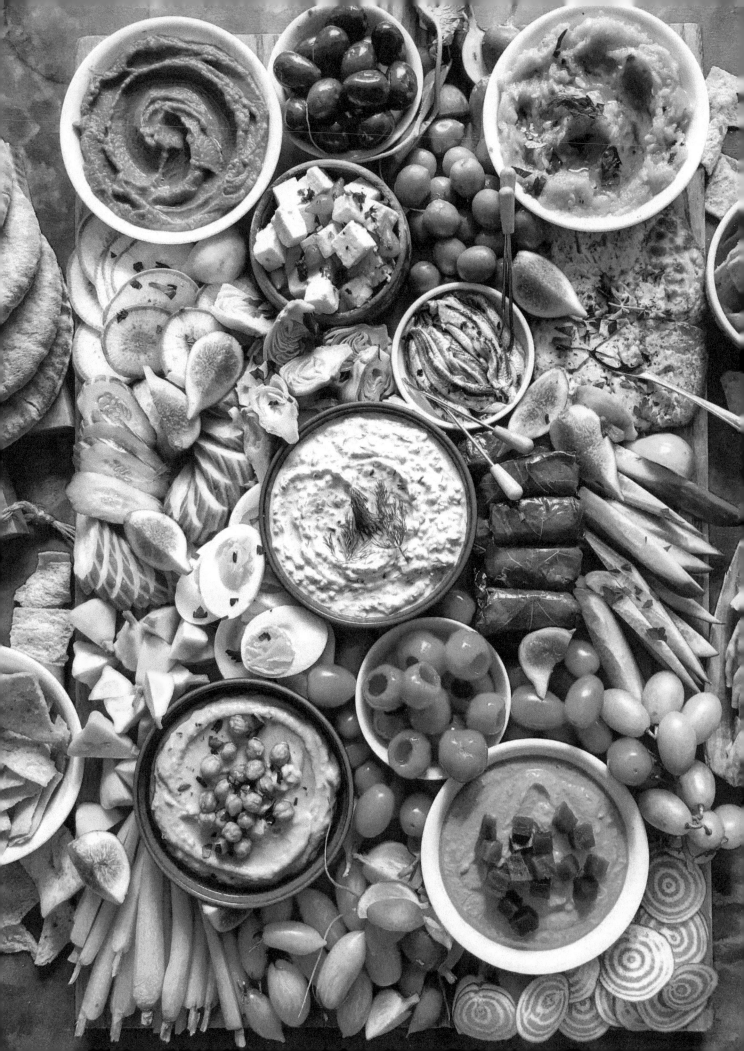

The Mediterranean Diet Cookbook for Beginners

1000 Easy, Healthy, and Flavorful Mediterranean Recipes for Everyday Cooking | 4-Week Meal Plan to Jumpstart Your Journey to Lifelong Health

Christy Thayer

CONTENT

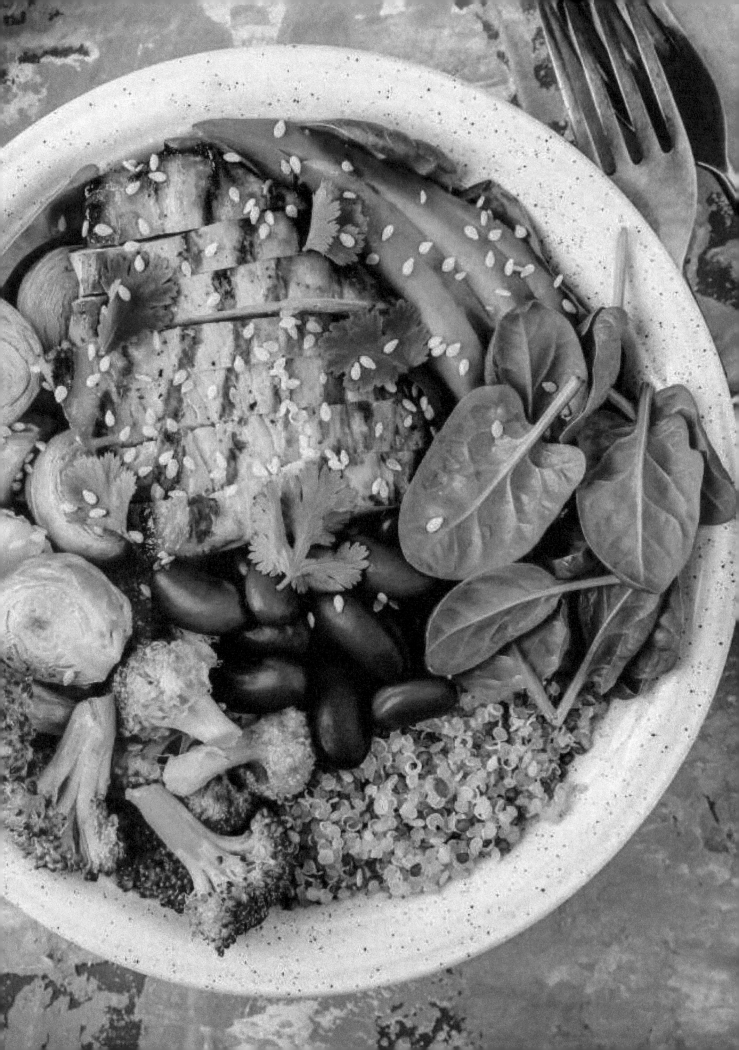

Introduction

The Mediterranean diet is fast becoming popular in the fitness world. This is because many people swear by it for its nutritional benefits and effectiveness. People who previously had difficulty adhering to other diets find that it is easier to stick to this diet. This is because the Mediterranean diet is not restrictive like other diets. It does not exclude any food group on the food pyramid; therefore, this makes it an all-around nutritional diet. Your body will not feel like it is starving on this diet.

Another great thing about it is that you do not have to count calories to lose weight. If you have been eating a high-calorie diet and have been carrying excess weight, you can expect to lose weight without starving yourself. But the craze is not just around the diet's effectiveness in weight loss. People are appreciating it for changing their eating habits and retraining their taste buds to appreciate food in its natural flavors. This book is all you need when it comes to understanding the Mediterranean diet. It tackles topics such as increasing longevity with the diet, as well as tackling health problems like heart disease and strokes. You will appreciate finding a summary of tips you will need to keep you on the diet as well as a few frequently asked questions answered. Go ahead and indulge in this lovely book, made just for you.

Chapter 1: The Basics of the Mediterranean Diet

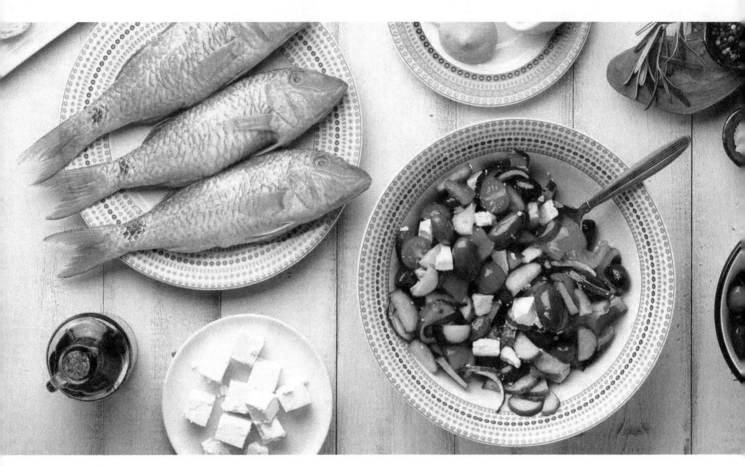

What Is the Mediterranean Diet?

Unlike some diets, the Mediterranean diet is relatively easy to adopt. This is because it is not too restrictive. This diet is based on the traditional diet of people who live around the Mediterranean sea, like from Italy, Spain, Greece, and Croatia. It is a diet that people naturally survived on and enjoyed. Therefore, it is not restrictive in the sense it follows an eating plan that people have lived on. Unlike some diets that people create, this diet has stood the test of time. It can easily be seen as a change in eating lifestyle. Not only is it healthy, but it is also delicious, as it offers a variety of tasty foods that you can nibble on. You will not feel like you are missing out on taste when you are on this diet because you are allowed to eat an array of plants and meats that all have different flavors. It has been recommended by dieticians for improving heart health as it is plant-based and rich in healthy fats like olive oil and omega-3 fatty acids from fish. With this diet, the more colorful your plate looks, the better (Gunnars, 2018).

The History of the Mediterranean Diet

The diet originates from areas within the Mediterranean basin. A detailed history of this diet is still unknown, however, understanding the ancient lifestyle of the people in that region helps us understand why the Mediterranean diet came to be. A large number of people in that area survived off of the foods that they farmed off their lands. These farms were rich in harvests of fruits and vegetables. As a result, fruits and vegetables became the staple foods of the area. Also, because they lived near the sea, fishing became something that most men in their communities did (Mayo Clinic Staff, 2019).

Men would frequently go out to catch fish for their households, which would then be eaten with the plants from the farm harvest. Cows were not common in the area, which meant that dairy and beef were also things that were not easily accessible to them. The climate in the area made it close to impossible for cows to live there because there would not be suitable grass for grazing. Protein was mostly acquired from fish, goats, and lamb. People who enjoy this diet appreciate it for its emphasis on natural flavors. When you are on it, your taste buds will be awakened and you will experience food as you have never done before.

The Scientific Value of the Mediterranean Diet

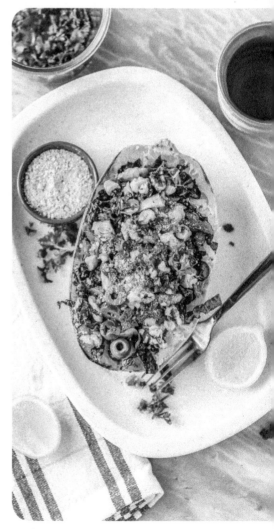

The Mediterranean diet is called the "heart-healthy" diet for a reason. This diet is rich in everything the doctor orders for your heart and anything you can think of. It is high in plant-based vitamins and minerals because it recommends the consumption of fresh fruits and vegetables, cereals, and legumes. The diet also recommends moderate amounts of fish and dairy and a limited amount of meat, saturated fats, and sugar. It is rich in healthy fats which usually come from nuts, olive oil, fatty fish, and seeds. Alcohol is recommended in moderation in the form of red wine (Mayo Clinic Staff, 2019).

Scientific research from the 1960s revealed that men who followed this diet were less likely to experience heart attacks. Similar research revealed that the Mediterranean diet lowers one's incidences of stroke, type 2 diabetes, and other cardiovascular diseases. Adherence to this diet has also been found to improve one's cognitive abilities. The antioxidants from all the fruits and vegetables as well as the red wine help reduce one's chances of getting Alzheimer's disease. Inflammation is the root cause of Alzheimer's disease and this diet's anti-inflammatory properties ensure that one is guarded against the disease. The brain also needs protein to sustain brain cells, which the diet offers in adequate amounts (Mayo Clinic Staff, 2019).

Chapter 2: The Benefits of Persisting the Mediterranean Diet

Increasing Longevity

The Mediterranean diet is a fountain of youth. The health benefits of this diet ensure that you will not develop any lifestyle diseases like heart disease, cancer, type 2 diabetes, and many more. The diet works with your body, for your body. When on this diet, you will be providing your body with the essential nutrients and minerals it craves when you are surviving on junk food. This diet will not only ensure that you shed some weight, but it will help you feel more alive as your energy levels will increase. Embark upon this new journey of health. Try it for a month and see how it goes. You will want to extend your period as you will appreciate the way your body will start to feel and the way your skin will start to look.

This diet is what your body has always been waiting for. What is even better with it is that you will not get tired of it like you would with low-carb and low-calorie diets. A great amount of research has been made that has found that this diet can be the solution to combating lifestyle diseases. If you are approaching senior years and you have been relatively healthy for all your life, this is also for you. Prevention is better than cure; it is best to start eating for your health now so that you do not regret it later (Mayo Clinic Staff, 2019).

Preventing Heart Disease and Strokes

Currently, the best treatment of heart disease and stroke is prevention. The Mediterranean diet can help you prevent both heart disease and strokes. For heart health, the key ingredient is in the healthy fats that the diet contains. The diet recommends that a person should drizzle olive oil over vegetables. Olive oil contains alpha-linolenic acid which has been found to reduce the risk of deaths in people with cardiovascular problems. Another source of healthy oil in the diet is fish. Fish is rich in omega-3 fatty acids which have been found to reduce cholesterol levels and lower blood pressure. This has been found to reduce mortality in cardiovascular disease patients (Mayo Clinic Staff, 2019).

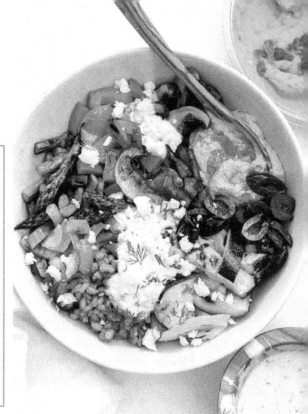

Weight Loss

If you have been falling on and off countless diets because they were just too hard to adhere to, this is the diet for you. Do you want to lose weight and keep it off without a hassle? As I have previously mentioned, the Mediterranean diet is more of an eating lifestyle change than it is a restrictive diet. You will lose weight when you are on this diet. Many people have expressed success with this diet, saying that it is easier to adhere to. However, the greatest benefit is that the diet not only gets you to lose weight but because you are eating healthier, you are guaranteed that you will feel healthier. The key is in the absence of processed foods and unhealthy fats. Another great thing about this diet is that you are welcome to alter it however you would rather prefer it. If you are not a fan of carbs, for instance, you can make this diet low carb by reducing your carb intake. You can also make it low protein if you want. The key focus is to make sure that you are eating plenty of fruits and vegetables. You will be more successful at this diet if you make it your own. Experiment in flavors in the first few weeks, but if you do not like them, feel free to make it your own by going for vegetables you would normally like.

Chapter 3: How to Stay on the Mediterranean Diet

If you are going to be successful on this diet, you will need to plan. Failure to plan is planning to fail. You need to have a clear plan that will guide you going forward. Ask yourself why you are adopting the diet; what is it that you want to achieve? Then you will need to write these goals down somewhere in reach. Determine what you would want to get out of the diet. Is it weight loss? Overall health? Prevention of illness? Whatever it is, write it down. If you write down your goals, you will be encouraged to move forward when you achieve even a little bit. However, be careful to set realistic and achievable goals for yourself. Yes, ideally you would want to attain great leaps of success, but the best way to plan is to take small steps toward your goal. Then you would need to commit each day of your week to do something toward reaching that goal. Set a reminder on your phone if you have to. Maybe organize the times you prepare your daily meals on a to-do list with alarm reminders to remind you to put some fresh vegetables into your meals and some fruits with your breakfast. No matter what, remember not to quit. Even if you fail on one day, bounce up and commit to the diet again the next day or two days later. Have a plan A, ask yourself what it would take to make the diet a delicious experience for you. If Plan A fails, then go for Plan B. Maybe make Plan A stricter than Plan B.

Take It Slow

Start slow if you have to. There is no rush, and you are likely to enjoy the diet if you ease into it. I know you may want to go into it headfirst. It is perfectly okay to try it that way, but if you know that you have had a lot of failures with previous diets, I recommend that you take it slowly. Consider replacing a large portion of your plate with vegetables instead of rice, then alternate days. Have a Mediterranean meal one day and your normal meal on the next. Introduce eating fruits with your cereals. Maybe add some berries or bananas to your oatmeal in the morning. These small steps are here to introduce your tastebuds to a new way of eating. Really, it is to gradually change your mindset around food. If you do not rush yourself, you will find that you will crave the Mediterranean dishes, which is the plan. You can start by enjoying smoothies and shakes. Just make sure that you do not make them too sweet. Try to enjoy your meals at their natural taste. It is a refreshing experience once you get used to it. Remember not to weigh your success by just weight loss. Remember that you undertaking this diet is a healthy lifestyle change and it is a success on its own. Also, even if you cheat for a day or two, you are doing well still because you go back to the diet. If you compare your diet before the Mediterranean diet, you will understand what I am saying. You are doing far better falling on and off it than you would be if you were eating how you used to.

Compare the Mediterranean Diet With the Food Pyramid

The Mediterranean diet emphasizes a lot of foods that are already on the food pyramid. It emphasizes vegetables, fruits, legumes, whole grains, olive oil. natural herbs and spices. For meat, it emphasizes fish, shellfish, poultry, and red meat in moderation. Eggs can also be eaten, as well as cheese and yogurt. Red wine is also fine in moderation. Compared to the food pyramid, the Mediterranean diet has smaller amounts of red meat and sweet fruits and has much healthier fats and oils. You can say that it does not go far off from the food pyramid. It honors the pyramid in every way except sizes (Gunnars, 2018).

The Mediterranean food pyramid differs from the conventional food pyramid. It emphasizes physical activity and enjoying your meals with the people you love. It also places emphasis on drinking water. It is recommended that you base all your daily meals on the second level of the pyramid which contains vegetables, fruits, legumes, whole grains, nuts and seeds, and beans (Gunnars, 2018).

Know the Difference Between Healthy and Unhealthy Fats

There are different types of fats found in foods grouped under monounsaturated, polyunsaturated, saturated, and trans fats.

Monounsaturated fats are a part of healthy fats. These are the fats that can be found in olives, avocados, nuts, and sunflower seeds.

Polyunsaturated fats are also healthy fats. These can be found in soybean, sunflower, corn, and safflower oils. They are good in aiding heart health as they lower bad cholesterol levels.

Saturated and trans fats should be your enemies. These are unhealthy fats that you should keep away from. Overconsumption of these fats can lead to serious complications. They increase your chances of getting cardiovascular illnesses and elevate bad cholesterol levels (Pasquale, 2017).

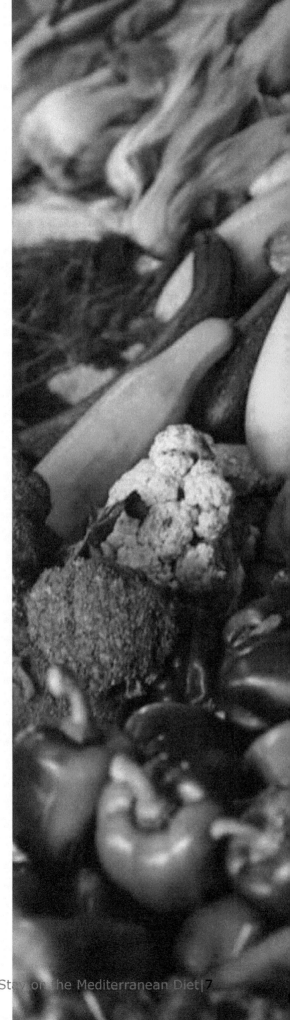

Chapter 4: The Mediterranean Lifestyle

You need to make sure that you have plenty of vegetables on your plate with every meal. Also, make sure that all the unhealthy foods that should not be eaten on the diet are not in your pantry or fridge. This will help you a lot because after all, you cannot eat what is not in your house.

The majority of your plate should be filled with fruits and vegetables. You should eat fish for about two or three days a week and eat red meat in moderation. Be careful not to neglect whole grains and legumes—these are packed with nutrients that will help you get the most out of the diet. Snack on nuts and seeds—they are tasty. Find the kinds you like and spoil yourself. You should also remember to cook your meals with olive oil and drink eight glasses of water a day with the occasional red wine glass (Gunnars, 2018).

Mediterranean Shopping Guide

Below is a list of items you should include on your Mediterranean diet shopping list (Gunnars, 2018):

- **Fruits:** Grapes, apples, berries, citrus fruits, avocados, bananas, papayas, pineapple, etc.
- **Frozen vegetables:** Healthy mixed veggie options
- **Vegetables:** Broccoli, mushrooms, celery, carrots, kale, onions, leeks, eggplant, etc.
- **Grains:** All whole grains including whole grain pasta and whole grain bread

- **Legumes:** Beans, lentils, peas, etc.
- **Seeds:** Pumpkin, hemp, sesame, sunflower, etc.
- **Nuts:** Almonds, walnuts, cashews, hazelnuts, pistachios, pine nuts, etc.
- Shellfish varieties and shrimp
- **Fish:** Salmon, tuna, herring, sardines, sea bass, etc.
- Baby potatoes and sweet potatoes

- Free-range chicken
- Natural Greek yogurt
- Cheese
- Pastured eggs
- Olives
- Extra-virgin olive oil
- **Meat:** goat, pork, and pastured beef

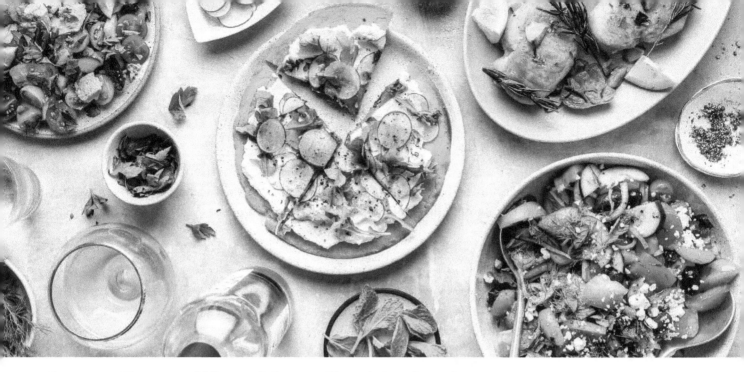

Ingredients That Must Be Limited

Below are foods and ingredients that should be limited or avoided while on the Mediterranean diet (Gunnars, 2018):

Heavily Processed Foods

In reality, everything has been processed. Even olive oil has been processed. However, some things are heavily processed. Things like frozen meals (which are high in sodium), sodas, candy, and desserts are so heavily processed that they lose their nutritional value.

Processed Red Meat

Here, I am talking about those hot dogs and that bacon we love. These are heavily processed and should be avoided at all costs. If you are having breakfast and you would like to have some meat included, opt to grill fresh meat like chicken from your fridge.

Refined Grains

Whole grains are emphasized in the Mediterranean diet; however, you should stay away from refined grains like white pasta and white bread.

Butter

Try replacing butter with olive oil. Butter has a lot of saturated fats that are bad for heart health.

Alcohol

The only alcohol allowed with this diet is red wine and that should be in moderation.

Eating Out on the Mediterranean Diet

The key to eating out when you are on the Mediterranean diet is to make sure that you do not stray from the diet. You will need to go to restaurants that can cater to your specifications. To be specific, you need to go to a place that offers fish, seafood, and vegetables. Ask the chef to fry your vegetables in extra virgin olive oil. And when you are eating bread, try not to spread it with butter, but ask for olive oil to dip in instead. For dessert, you can enjoy a glass of red wine with some fruits like grapes or berries, maybe even with a dash of Greek yogurt (Gunnars, 2018).

Questions & Answers

Does the Mediterranean Diet Let Me Eat Carbs?

The Mediterranean diet does not cut out any food group or macronutrient. However, you need to be wise about the kind of carbohydrates you put in your mouth. I think you can agree that eating chips as a form of carbohydrates is not a good idea. Of course, you can eat brown rice, brown pasta, etc.

Can I Still Eat Dessert?

The good news is yes, you can. However, you need to make sure that you eat desserts in moderation. The key is to keep your eye on your sugar intake. Also, you can always opt for sweet fruits with Greek yogurt for dessert.

Is the Mediterranean Diet Expensive?

If you consider that you will mainly be eating fresh produce, beans, and whole grains with not too much meat, I say no. This diet is not expensive. If you compare it to other diets which cut out some food groups and those that focus on protein, you are likely to save a lot of money on this diet. Another thing is you will not be eating out as much as you used to.

Will I Lose Weight on the Mediterranean Diet?

Yes, if you are carrying some excess weight, you will shed some weight. There is no need to count calories on this diet. However, if you have been eating a high-calorie diet, the Mediterranean diet will have you on a calorie deficit which will make you lose weight. Another thing to consider is that this diet is nutrient filled so you will feel full longer.

Can I Still Drink Coffee?

Drinking coffee is allowed on this diet. Again, you need to keep your eyes on your sugar intake. If you are used to getting your coffee at a coffee shop, for instance, try to opt for a sugar-free one.

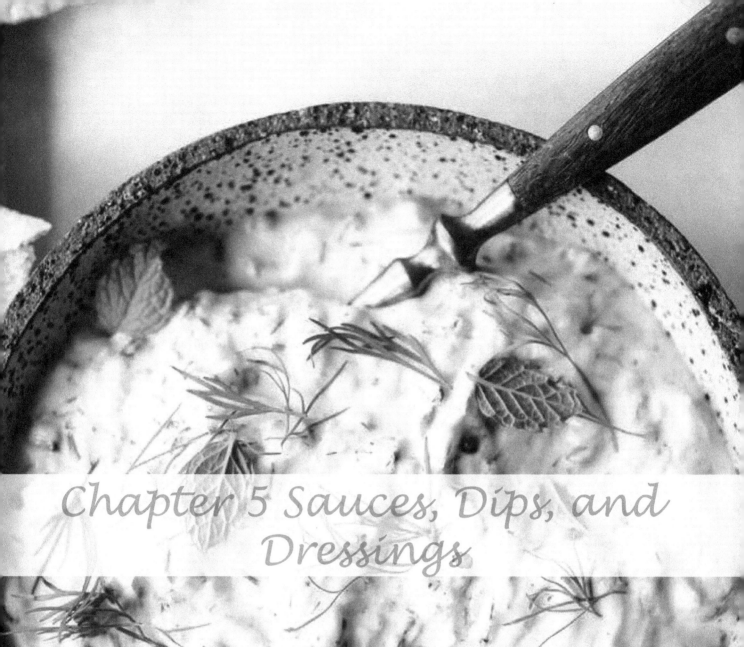
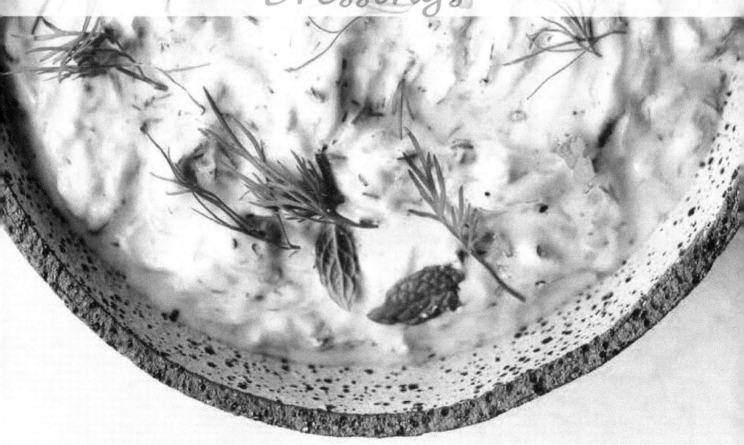

Chapter 5 Sauces, Dips, and Dressings

Oregano Cucumber Dressing

Prep time: 5 minutes | Cook time: 0 minutes | Serves 2

1½ cups plain, unsweetened, full-fat Greek yogurt
1 cucumber, seeded and peeled
½ lemon, juiced and zested
1 tablespoon dried, minced garlic
½ tablespoon dried dill
2 teaspoons dried oregano
Salt, to taste

1. In a food processor, combine the yogurt, cucumber, lemon juice, garlic, dill, oregano, and a pinch of salt and process until smooth. Adjust the seasonings as needed and transfer to a serving bowl.

Per Serving
calories: 209 | fat: 10g | protein: 18g
carbs: 14g | fiber: 2g | sodium: 69mg

Fresh Herb Butter

Prep time: 5 minutes | Cook time: 0 minutes | Makes ½ cup

½ cup almond butter, at room temperature
1 garlic clove, finely minced
2 teaspoons finely chopped fresh
rosemary
1 teaspoon finely chopped fresh oregano
½ teaspoon salt

1. In a food processor, combine the almond butter, garlic, rosemary, oregano, and salt and pulse until the mixture is well combined, smooth, and creamy, scraping down the sides as necessary. Alternatively, you can whip the ingredients together with an electric mixer.
2. Using a spatula, scrape the almond butter mixture into a small bowl or glass container and cover. Store in the refrigerator for up to 1 month.

Per Serving (1 tablespoon)
calories: 103 | fat: 12g | protein: 0g
carbs: 0g | fiber: 0g | sodium: 227mg

Tarragon Grapefruit Dressing

Prep time: 5 minutes | Cook time: 0 minutes | Serves 4 to 6

½ cup avocado oil mayonnaise
2 tablespoons Dijon mustard
1 teaspoon dried tarragon or 1 tablespoon chopped fresh tarragon
Zest and juice of ½ grapefruit (about 2 tablespoons juice)
½ teaspoon salt
¼ teaspoon freshly ground black pepper
1 to 2 tablespoons water (optional)

1. In a large mason jar or glass measuring cup, combine the mayonnaise, Dijon, tarragon, grapefruit zest and juice, salt, and pepper and whisk well with a fork until smooth and creamy. If a thinner dressing is preferred, thin out with water.

Per Serving (2 tablespoons)
calories: 86 | fat: 7g | protein: 1g
carbs: 6g | fiber: 0g | sodium: 390mg

Oregano Cucumber Dressing

Prep time: 5 minutes | Cook time: 0 minutes | Serves 2

1½ cups plain, unsweetened, full-fat Greek yogurt
1 cucumber, seeded and peeled
½ lemon, juiced and zested
1 tablespoon dried, minced garlic
½ tablespoon dried dill
2 teaspoons dried oregano
Salt, to taste

1. In a food processor, combine the yogurt, cucumber, lemon juice, garlic, dill, oregano, and a pinch of salt and process until smooth. Adjust the seasonings as needed and transfer to a serving bowl.

Per Serving
calories: 209 | fat: 10g | protein: 18g
carbs: 14g | fiber: 2g | sodium: 69mg

Bagna Cauda
Prep time: 5 minutes | Cook time: 20 minutes | Serves 8 to 10

½ cup extra-virgin olive oil
4 tablespoons (½ stick) butter (optional)
8 anchovy fillets, very finely chopped
4 large garlic cloves, finely minced
½ teaspoon salt
½ teaspoon freshly ground black pepper

1. In a small saucepan, heat the olive oil and butter (if desired) over medium-low heat until the butter is melted.
2. Add the anchovies and garlic and stir to combine. Add the salt and pepper and reduce the heat to low. Cook, stirring occasionally, until the anchovies are very soft and the mixture is very fragrant, about 20 minutes.
3. Serve warm, drizzled over steamed vegetables, as a dipping sauce for raw veggies or cooked artichokes, or use as a salad dressing. Store leftovers in an airtight container in the refrigerator for up to 2 weeks.

Per Serving (2 tablespoons)
calories: 181 | fat: 20g | protein: 1g
carbs: 1g | fiber: 0g | sodium: 333mg

Tahini Dressing
Prep time: 5 minutes | Cook time: 0 minutes | Serves 8 to 10

½ cup tahini
¼ cup freshly squeezed lemon juice (about 2 to 3 lemons)
¼ cup extra-virgin olive oil
1 garlic clove, finely minced or ½ teaspoon garlic powder
2 teaspoons salt

1. In a glass mason jar with a lid, combine the tahini, lemon juice, olive oil, garlic, and salt. Cover and shake well until combined and creamy. Store in the refrigerator for up to 2 weeks.

Per Serving (2 tablespoons)
calories: 121 | fat: 12g | protein: 2g
carbs: 2g | fiber: 1g | sodium: 479mg

Easy Tzatziki Sauce
Prep time: 5 minutes | Cook time: 0 minutes | Serves 2

1 medium cucumber, peeled, seeded and diced
½ teaspoon salt, divided, plus more
½ cup plain, unsweetened, full-fat Greek yogurt
½ lemon, juiced
1 tablespoon chopped fresh parsley
½ teaspoon dried minced garlic
½ teaspoon dried dill
Freshly ground black pepper, to taste

1. Put the cucumber in a colander. Sprinkle with ¼ teaspoon of salt and toss. Let the cucumber rest at room temperature in the colander for 30 minutes.
2. Rinse the cucumber in cool water and place in a single layer on several layers of paper towels to remove the excess liquid.
3. In a food processor, pulse the cucumber to chop finely and drain off any extra fluid.
4. Pour the cucumber into a mixing bowl and add the yogurt, lemon juice, parsley, garlic, dill, and the remaining ¼ teaspoon of salt. Season with salt and pepper to taste and whisk the ingredients together. Refrigerate in an airtight container.

Per Serving
calories: 77 | fat: 3g | protein: 6g
carbs: 6g | fiber: 1g | sodium: 607mg

Apple Cider Dressing
Prep time: 5 minutes | Cook time: 0 minutes | Serves 2

2 tablespoons apple cider vinegar
1/3 lemon, juiced
1/3 lemon, zested
Salt and freshly ground black pepper, to taste

1. In a jar, combine the vinegar, lemon juice, and zest. Season with salt and pepper, cover, and shake well.

Per Serving
calories: 4 | fat: 0g | protein: 0g
carbs: 1g | fiber: 0g | sodium: 0mg

Cucumber Yogurt Dip

Prep time: 5 minutes | Cook time: 0 minutes | Serves 2 to 3

1 cup plain, unsweetened, full-fat Greek yogurt
½ cup cucumber, peeled, seeded, and diced
1 tablespoon freshly squeezed lemon juice
1 tablespoon chopped fresh mint
1 small garlic clove, minced
Salt and freshly ground black pepper, to taste

1. In a food processor, combine the yogurt, cucumber, lemon juice, mint, and garlic. Pulse several times to combine, leaving noticeable cucumber chunks.
2. Taste and season with salt and pepper.

Per Serving
calories: 128 | fat: 6g | protein: 11g
carbs: 7g | fiber: 0g | sodium: 47mg

Orange Dijon Dressing

Prep time: 5 minutes | Cook time: 0 minutes | Serves 2

¼ cup extra-virgin olive oil
2 tablespoons freshly squeezed orange juice
1 orange, zested
1 teaspoon garlic powder
¾ teaspoon za'atar seasoning
½ teaspoon salt
¼ teaspoon Dijon mustard
Freshly ground black pepper, to taste

1. In a jar, combine the olive oil, orange juice and zest, garlic powder, za'atar, salt, and mustard. Season with pepper and shake vigorously until completely mixed.

Per Serving
calories: 283 | fat: 27g | protein: 1g
carbs: 11g | fiber:2 g | sodium: 597mg

Creamy Yogurt Dressing

Prep time: 5 minutes | Cook time: 0 minutes | Serves 3

1 cup plain, unsweetened, full-fat Greek yogurt
½ cup extra-virgin olive oil
1 tablespoon apple cider vinegar
½ lemon, juiced
1 tablespoon chopped fresh oregano
½ teaspoon dried parsley
½ teaspoon kosher salt
¼ teaspoon garlic powder
¼ teaspoon freshly ground black pepper

1. In a large bowl, combine the yogurt, olive oil, vinegar, lemon juice, oregano, parsley, salt, garlic powder, and pepper and whisk well.

Per Serving
calories: 402 | fat: 40g | protein: 8g
carbs: 4g | fiber: 0g | sodium: 417mg

Arugula Walnut Pesto

Prep time: 5 minutes | Cook time: 0 minutes | Serves 8 to 10

6 cups packed arugula
1 cup chopped walnuts
½ cup shredded Parmesan cheese
2 garlic cloves, peeled
½ teaspoon salt
1 cup extra-virgin olive oil

1. In a food processor, combine the arugula, walnuts, cheese, and garlic and process until very finely chopped. Add the salt. With the processor running, stream in the olive oil until well blended.
2. If the mixture seems too thick, add warm water, 1 tablespoon at a time, until smooth and creamy. Store in a sealed container in the refrigerator.

Per Serving (2 tablespoons)
calories: 296 | fat: 31g | protein: 4g
carbs: 2g | fiber: 1g | sodium: 206mg

Red Wine Vinaigrette

Prep time: 5 minutes | Cook time: 0 minutes | Serves 2

¼ cup plus 2 tablespoons extra-virgin olive oil
2 tablespoons red wine vinegar
1 tablespoon apple cider vinegar
2 teaspoons honey

2 teaspoons Dijon mustard
½ teaspoon minced garlic
⅛ teaspoon kosher salt
⅛ teaspoon freshly ground black pepper

1. In a jar, combine the olive oil, vinegars, honey, mustard, garlic, salt, and pepper and shake well.

Per Serving
calories: 386 | fat: 41g | protein: 0g
carbs: 6g | fiber: 0g | sodium: 198mg

Marinara Sauce

Prep time: 15 minutes | Cook time: 40 minutes | Makes 8 cups

1 small onion, diced
1 small red bell pepper, stemmed, seeded and chopped
2 tablespoons plus ¼ cup extra-virgin olive oil, divided
2 tablespoons butter (optional)
4 to 6 garlic cloves, minced
2 teaspoon salt, divided
½ teaspoon freshly

ground black pepper
2 (32-ounce / 907-g) cans crushed tomatoes (with basil, if possible), with their juices
½ cup thinly sliced basil leaves, divided
2 tablespoons chopped fresh rosemary
1 to 2 teaspoons crushed red pepper flakes (optional)

1. In a food processor, combine the onion and bell pepper and blend until very finely minced.
2. In a large skillet, heat 2 tablespoons olive oil and the butter (if desired) over medium heat. Add the minced onion, and red pepper and sauté until just starting to get tender, about 5 minutes.
3. Add the garlic, salt, and pepper and sauté until fragrant, another 1 to 2 minutes.

4. Reduce the heat to low and add the tomatoes and their juices, remaining ¼ cup olive oil, ¼ cup basil, rosemary, and red pepper flakes (if using). Stir to combine, then bring to a simmer and cover. Cook over low heat for 30 to 60 minutes to allow the flavors to blend.
5. Add remaining ¼ cup chopped fresh basil after removing from heat, stirring to combine.

Per Serving (1 cup)
calories: 256 | fat: 20g | protein: 4g
carbs: 19g | fiber: 5g | sodium: 803mg

Romesco Sauce

Prep time: 10 minutes | Cook time: 0 minutes | Serves 10

1 (12-ounce / 340-g) jar roasted red peppers, drained
1 (14½-ounce / 411-g) can diced tomatoes, undrained
½ cup dry-roasted almonds
2 garlic cloves
2 teaspoons red wine vinegar
1 teaspoon smoked paprika or ½ teaspoon cayenne pepper

¼ teaspoon kosher or sea salt
¼ teaspoon freshly ground black pepper
¼ cup extra-virgin olive oil
⅔ cup torn, day-old bread or toast
Assortment of sliced raw vegetables such as carrots, celery, cucumber, green beans, and bell peppers, for serving

1. In a high-powered blender or food processor, combine the roasted peppers, tomatoes and their juices, almonds, garlic, vinegar, smoked paprika, salt, and pepper.
2. Begin puréeing the ingredients on medium speed, and slowly drizzle in the oil with the blender running. Continue to purée until the dip is thoroughly mixed.
3. Add the bread and purée.
4. Serve with raw vegetables for dipping, or store in a jar with a lid for up to one week in the refrigerator.

Per Serving
calories: 96 | fat: 7g | protein: 3g
carbs: 8g | fiber: 3g | sodium: 2mg

Pineapple Salsa

Prep time: 10 minutes | Cook time: 0 minutes | Serves 6 to 8

1 pound (454 g) fresh or thawed frozen pineapple, finely diced, juices reserved
1 white or red onion, finely diced
1 bunch cilantro or mint, leaves only, chopped
1 jalapeño, minced (optional)
Salt, to taste

1. Stir together the pineapple with its juice, onion, cilantro, and jalapeño (if desired) in a medium bowl. Season with salt to taste and serve.
2. The salsa can be refrigerated in an airtight container for up to 2 days.

Per Serving
calories: 55 | fat: 0g | protein: 1g
carbs: 12g | fiber: 2g | sodium: 20mg

Spanakopita Dip

Prep time: 15 minutes | Cook time: 14 minutes | Serves 2

Olive oil cooking spray
3 tablespoons olive oil, divided
2 tablespoons minced white onion
2 garlic cloves, minced
4 cups fresh spinach
4 ounces (113 g) cream cheese, softened
4 ounces (113 g) feta cheese, divided
Zest of 1 lemon
¼ teaspoon ground nutmeg
1 teaspoon dried dill
½ teaspoon salt
Pita chips, carrot sticks, or sliced bread for serving (optional)

1. Preheat the air fryer to 360ºF (182ºC). Coat the inside of a 6-inch ramekin or baking dish with olive oil cooking spray.
2. In a large skillet over medium heat, heat 1 tablespoon of the olive oil. Add the onion, then cook for 1 minute.
3. Add in the garlic and cook, stirring for 1 minute more.
4. Reduce the heat to low and mix in the spinach and water. Let this cook for 2 to 3 minutes, or until the spinach has wilted. Remove the skillet from the heat.
5. In a medium bowl, combine the cream cheese, 2 ounces of the feta, and the remaining 2 tablespoons of olive oil, along with the lemon zest, nutmeg, dill, and salt. Mix until just combined.
6. Add the vegetables to the cheese base and stir until combined.
7. Pour the dip mixture into the prepared ramekin and top with the remaining 2 ounces of feta cheese.
8. Place the dip into the air fryer basket and cook for 10 minutes, or until heated through and bubbling.
9. Serve with pita chips, carrot sticks, or sliced bread.

Per Serving
calories: 550 | fat: 52g | protein: 14g
carbs: 9g | fiber: 2g | sodium: 113mg

Harissa Sauce

Prep time: 10 minutes | Cook time: 20 minutes | Makes 3 to 4 cups

1 large red bell pepper, deseeded, cored, and cut into chunks
1 yellow onion, cut into thick rings
4 garlic cloves, peeled
1 cup vegetable broth
2 tablespoons tomato paste
1 tablespoon tamari
1 teaspoon ground cumin
1 tablespoon Hungarian paprika

1. Preheat the oven to 450ºF (235ºC). Line a baking sheet with parchment paper.
2. Place the bell pepper on the prepared baking sheet, flesh-side up, and space out the onion and garlic around the pepper.
3. Roast in the preheated oven for 20 minutes. Transfer to a blender.
4. Add the vegetable broth, tomato paste, tamari, cumin, and paprika. Purée until smooth. Served chilled or warm.

Per Serving (¼ cup)
calories: 15 | fat: 1g | protein: 1g
carbs: 3g | fiber: 1g | sodium: 201mg

Rosemary Garlic Infused Olive Oil
Prep time: 5 minutes | Cook time: 30 minutes | Makes 1 cup

1 cup extra-virgin olive oil
4 large garlic cloves, smashed

4 (4- to 5-inch) sprigs rosemary

1. In a medium skillet, heat the olive oil, garlic, and rosemary sprigs over low heat. Cook until fragrant and garlic is very tender, 30 to 45 minutes, stirring occasionally. Don't let the oil get too hot or the garlic will burn and become bitter.
2. Remove from the heat and allow to cool slightly. Remove the garlic and rosemary with a slotted spoon and pour the oil into a glass container. Allow to cool completely before covering. Store covered at room temperature for up to 3 months.

Per Serving (2 tablespoons)
calories: 241 | fat: 26g | protein: 0g | carbs: 1g | fiber: 0g | sodium: 1mg

Pearl Onion Dip
Prep time: 10 minutes | Cook time: 12 minutes | Serves 4

2 cups peeled pearl onions
3 garlic cloves
3 tablespoons olive oil, divided
½ teaspoon salt
1 cup nonfat plain Greek yogurt

1 tablespoon lemon juice
¼ teaspoon black pepper
⅛ teaspoon red pepper flakes
Pita chips, vegetables, or toasted bread for serving (optional)

1. Preheat the air fryer to 360ºF (182ºC).
2. In a large bowl, combine the pearl onions and garlic with 2 tablespoons of the olive oil until the onions are well coated.
3. Pour the garlic-and-onion mixture into the air fryer basket and roast for 12 minutes.
4. Transfer the garlic and onions to a food processor. Pulse the vegetables several times, until the onions are minced but still have some chunks.
5. In a large bowl, combine the garlic and onions and the remaining 1 tablespoon of olive oil, along with the salt, yogurt, lemon juice, black pepper, and red pepper flakes.
6. Cover and chill for 1 hour before serving with pita chips, vegetables, or toasted bread.

Per Serving
calories: 150 | fat: 10g | protein: 7g | carbs: 7g | fiber: 1g | sodium: 3mg

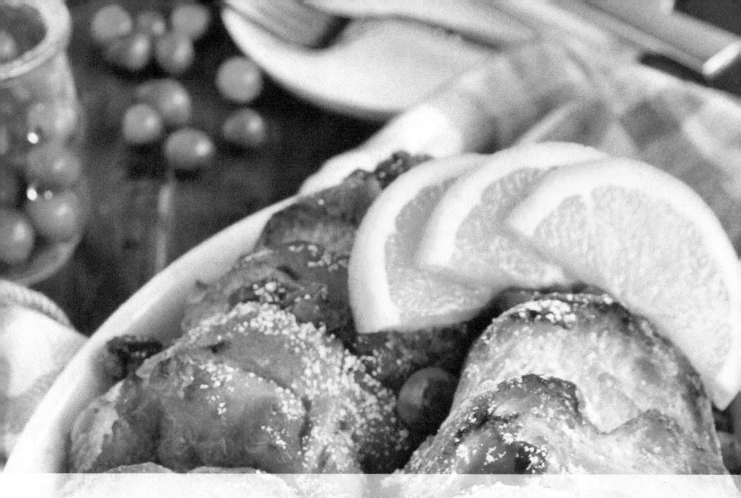
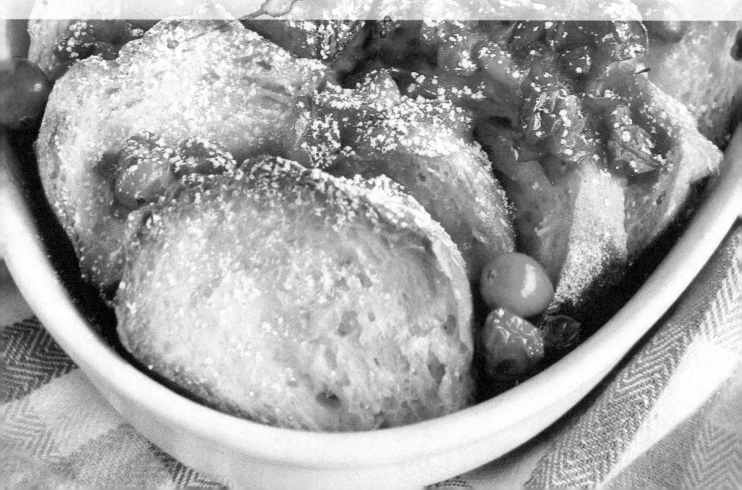

Chapter 6 Breakfasts

Orange French Toast

Prep time: 5 minutes | Cook time: 15 minutes | Serves 6

1 cup unsweetened almond milk
3 large eggs
2 teaspoons grated orange zest
1 teaspoon vanilla extract
⅛ teaspoon ground cardamom
⅛ teaspoon ground cinnamon
1 loaf of boule bread, sliced 1 inch thick (gluten-free preferred)
1 banana, sliced
¼ cup Berry and Honey Compote

1. Heat a large nonstick sauté pan or skillet over medium-high heat.
2. In a large, shallow dish, mix the milk, eggs, orange zest, vanilla, cardamom, and cinnamon. Working in batches, dredge the bread slices in the egg mixture and put in the hot pan.
3. Cook for 5 minutes on each side, until golden brown. Serve, topped with banana and drizzled with honey compote.

Per Serving
calories: 394 | fat: 6g | protein: 17g
carbs: 68g | fiber: 3g | sodium: 716mg

Greek Yogurt Parfait with Nuts

Prep time: 10 minutes | Cook time: 0 minutes | Serves 1

½ cup plain whole-milk Greek yogurt
2 tablespoons heavy whipping cream
¼ cup frozen berries, thawed with juices
½ teaspoon vanilla or almond extract
(optional)
¼ teaspoon ground cinnamon (optional)
1 tablespoon ground flaxseed
2 tablespoons chopped nuts (walnuts or pecans)

1. In a small bowl or glass, combine the yogurt, heavy whipping cream, thawed berries in their juice, vanilla or almond extract (if using), cinnamon (if using), and flaxseed and stir well until smooth. Top with chopped nuts and enjoy.

Per Serving
calories: 267 | fat: 19g | protein: 11g
carbs: 12g | fiber: 3g | sodium: 63mg

Sweet Potato Toast

Prep time: 5 minutes | Cook time: 1 minutes | Serves 4

2 plum tomatoes, halved
6 tablespoons extra-virgin olive oil, divided
Salt and freshly ground black pepper, to taste
2 large sweet potatoes, sliced lengthwise
1 cup fresh spinach
8 medium asparagus, trimmed
4 large cooked eggs or egg substitute (poached, scrambled, or fried)
1 cup arugula
4 tablespoons pesto
4 tablespoons shredded Asiago cheese

1. Preheat the oven to 450ºF (235ºC).
2. On a baking sheet, brush the plum tomato halves with 2 tablespoons of olive oil and season with salt and pepper. Roast the tomatoes in the oven for approximately 15 minutes, then remove from the oven and allow to rest.
3. Put the sweet potato slices on a separate baking sheet and brush about 2 tablespoons of oil on each side and season with salt and pepper. Bake the sweet potato slices for about 15 minutes, flipping once after 5 to 7 minutes, until just tender. Remove from the oven and set aside.
4. In a sauté pan or skillet, heat the remaining 2 tablespoons of olive oil over medium heat and sauté the fresh spinach until just wilted. Remove from the pan and rest on a paper towel-lined dish. In the same pan, add the asparagus and sauté, turning throughout. Transfer to a paper towel-lined dish.
5. Place the slices of grilled sweet potato on serving plates and divide the spinach and asparagus evenly among the slices. Place a prepared egg on top of the spinach and asparagus. Top this with ¼ cup of arugula.
6. Finish by drizzling with 1 tablespoon of pesto and sprinkle with 1 tablespoon of cheese. Serve with 1 roasted plum tomato.

Per Serving
calories: 441 | fat: 35g | protein: 13g
carbs: 23g | fiber: 4g | sodium: 481mg

Cheesy Mini Frittatas

Prep time: 10 minutes | Cook time: 25 minutes | Serves 6

Nonstick cooking spray
1½ tablespoons extra-virgin olive oil
¼ cup chopped red potatoes (about 3 small)
¼ cup minced onions
¼ cup chopped red bell pepper
¼ cup asparagus, sliced lengthwise in half and chopped
4 large eggs
4 large egg whites
½ cup unsweetened almond milk
Salt and freshly ground black pepper, to taste
½ cup shredded low-moisture, part-skim Mozzarella cheese, divided

1. Preheat the oven to 350ºF (180ºC). Using nonstick cooking spray, prepare a 12-count muffin pan.
2. In a medium sauté pan or skillet, heat the oil over medium heat and sauté the potatoes and onions for about 4 minutes, until the potatoes are fork-tender.
3. Add the bell pepper and asparagus and sauté for about 4 minutes, until just tender. Transfer the contents of a pan onto a paper-towel-lined plate to cool.
4. In a bowl, whisk together the eggs, egg whites, and milk. Season with salt and pepper.
5. Once the vegetables are cooled to room temperature, add the vegetables and ¼ cup of Mozzarella cheese.
6. Using a spoon or ladle, evenly distribute the contents of the bowl into the prepared muffin pan, filling the cups about halfway.
7. Sprinkle the remaining ¼ cup of cheese over the top of the cups.
8. Bake for 20 to 25 minutes, or until eggs reach an internal temperature of 145ºF (63ºC) or the center is solid.
9. Allow the mini frittatas to rest for 5 to 10 minutes before removing from muffin pan and serving.

Per Serving (2 mini frittatas)
calories: 133 | fat: 9g | protein: 10g
carbs: 4g | fiber: 1g | sodium: 151mg

Morning Creamy Iced Coffee

Prep time: 5 minutes | Cook time: 0 minutes | Serves 1

1 cup freshly brewed strong black coffee, cooled slightly
1 tablespoon extra-virgin olive oil
1 tablespoon half-and-half or heavy cream (optional)
1 teaspoon MCT oil (optional)
⅛ teaspoon almond extract
⅛ teaspoon ground cinnamon

1. Pour the slightly cooled coffee into a blender or large glass (if using an immersion blender).
2. Add the olive oil, half-and-half (if using), MCT oil (if using), almond extract, and cinnamon.
3. Blend well until smooth and creamy. Drink warm and enjoy.

Per Serving
calories: 128 | fat: 14g | protein: 0g
carbs: 0g | fiber: 0g | sodium: 5mg

Pumpkin Layers with Honey Granola

Prep time: 5 minutes | Cook time: 0 minutes | Serves 4

1 (15-ounce / 425-g) can pure pumpkin purée
4 teaspoons honey, additional to taste
1 teaspoon pumpkin pie spice
¼ teaspoon ground cinnamon
2 cups plain, unsweetened, full-fat Greek yogurt
1 cup honey granola

1. In a large bowl, mix the pumpkin purée, honey, pumpkin pie spice, and cinnamon. Cover and refrigerate for at least 2 hours.
2. To make the parfaits, in each cup, pour ¼ cup pumpkin mix, ¼ cup yogurt and ¼ cup granola. Repeat Greek yogurt and pumpkin layers and top with honey granola.

Per Serving
calories: 264 | fat: 9g | protein: 15g
carbs: 35g | fiber: 6g | sodium: 90mg

Cardamom-Cinnamon Overnight Oats

Prep time: 10 minutes | Cook time: 0 minutes | Serves 2

½ cup vanilla, unsweetened almond milk (not Silk brand)
½ cup rolled oats
2 tablespoons sliced almonds
2 tablespoons simple sugar liquid sweetener
1 teaspoon chia seeds
¼ teaspoon ground cardamom
¼ teaspoon ground cinnamon

1. In a mason jar, combine the almond milk, oats, almonds, liquid sweetener, chia seeds, cardamom, and cinnamon and shake well. Store in the refrigerator for 8 to 24 hours, then serve cold or heated.

Per Serving
calories: 131 | fat: 6g | protein: 5g
carbs: 17g | fiber: 4g | sodium: 45mg

Blueberry and Chia Seeds Smoothie

Prep time: 10 minutes | Cook time: 0 minutes | Serves 1

1 cup unsweetened almond milk, plus more as needed
¼ cup frozen blueberries
2 tablespoons unsweetened almond butter
1 tablespoon ground flaxseed or chia seeds
1 tablespoon extra-virgin olive oil or avocado oil
1 to 2 teaspoons stevia or monk fruit extract (optional)
½ teaspoon vanilla extract
¼ teaspoon ground cinnamon

1. In a blender or a large wide-mouth jar, if using an immersion blender, combine the almond milk, blueberries, almond butter, flaxseed, olive oil, stevia (if using), vanilla, and cinnamon and blend until smooth and creamy, adding more almond milk to achieve your desired consistency.

Per Serving
calories: 460 | fat: 40g | protein: 8g
carbs: 20g | fiber: 9g | sodium: 147mg

Versatile Sandwich Round

Prep time: 5 minutes | Cook time: 2 minutes | Serves 1

3 tablespoons almond flour
1 tablespoon extra-virgin olive oil
1 large egg
½ teaspoon dried rosemary, oregano, basil, thyme, or garlic powder (optional)
¼ teaspoon baking powder
⅛ teaspoon salt

1. In a microwave-safe ramekin, combine the almond flour, olive oil, egg, rosemary (if using), baking powder, and salt. Mix well with a fork.
2. Microwave for 90 seconds on high.
3. Slide a knife around the edges of ramekin and flip to remove the bread.
4. Slice in half with a serrated knife if you want to use it to make a sandwich.

Per Serving
calories: 232 | fat: 22g | protein: 8g
carbs: 1g | fiber: 0g | sodium: 450mg

Banana Corn Fritters

Prep time: 5 minutes | Cook time: 10 minutes | Serves 2

½ cup yellow cornmeal
¼ cup flour
2 small ripe bananas, peeled and mashed
2 tablespoons unsweetened almond milk
1 large egg, beaten
½ teaspoon baking powder
¼ to ½ teaspoon ground chipotle chili
¼ teaspoon ground cinnamon
¼ teaspoon sea salt
1 tablespoon olive oil

1. Stir together all ingredients except for the olive oil in a large bowl until smooth.
2. Heat a nonstick skillet over medium-high heat. Add the olive oil and drop about 2 tablespoons of batter for each fritter. Cook for 2 to 3 minutes until the bottoms are golden brown, then flip. Continue cooking for 1 to 2 minutes more, until cooked through. Repeat with the remaining batter.
3. Serve warm.

Per Serving
calories: 396 | fat: 10g | protein: 7g
carbs: 68g | fiber: 4g | sodium: 307mg

Avocado Toast with Poached Eggs

Prep time: 5 minutes | Cook time: 7 minutes | Serves 4

Olive oil cooking spray	4 pieces whole grain bread
4 large eggs	1 avocado
Salt and black pepper, to taste	Red pepper flakes (optional)

1. Preheat the air fryer to 320ºF (160ºC). Lightly coat the inside of four small oven-safe ramekins with olive oil cooking spray.
2. Crack one egg into each ramekin, and season with salt and black pepper.
3. Place the ramekins into the air fryer basket. Close and set the timer to 7 minutes.
4. While the eggs are cooking, toast the bread in a toaster.
5. Slice the avocado in half lengthwise, remove the pit, and scoop the flesh into a small bowl. Season with salt, black pepper, and red pepper flakes, if desired. Using a fork, smash the avocado lightly.
6. Spread a quarter of the smashed avocado evenly over each slice of toast.
7. Remove the eggs from the air fryer, and gently spoon one onto each slice of avocado toast before serving.

Per Serving
calories: 232 | fat: 14g | protein: 11g
carbs: 18g | fiber: 6g | sodium: 175mg

Prosciutto, Avocado, and Veggie Sandwiches

Prep time: 10 minutes | Cook time: 0 minutes | Serves 4

8 slices whole-grain or whole-wheat bread	4 romaine lettuce leaves, torn into 8 pieces total
1 ripe avocado, halved and pitted	1 large, ripe tomato, sliced into 8 rounds
¼ teaspoon freshly ground black pepper	2 ounces (57 g) prosciutto, cut into 8 thin slices
¼ teaspoon kosher or sea salt	

1. Toast the bread and place on a large platter.

2. Scoop the avocado flesh out of the skin into a small bowl. Add the pepper and salt. Using a fork or a whisk, gently mash the avocado until it resembles a creamy spread. Spread the avocado mash over all 8 pieces of toast.
3. To make one sandwich, take one slice of avocado toast, and top it with a lettuce leaf, tomato slice, and prosciutto slice. Top with another slice each of lettuce, tomato, and prosciutto, then cover with a second piece of avocado toast (avocado-side down on the prosciutto). Repeat with the remaining ingredients to make three more sandwiches and serve.

Per Serving
calories: 262 | fat: 12g | protein: 8g
carbs: 35g | fiber: 10g | sodium: 162mg

Feta and Pepper Frittata

Prep time: 10 minutes | Cook time: 20 minutes | Serves 4

Olive oil cooking spray	½ teaspoon salt
8 large eggs	½ teaspoon black pepper
1 medium red bell pepper, diced	1 garlic clove, minced
	½ cup feta, divided

1. Preheat the air fryer to 360ºF (182ºC). Lightly coat the inside of a 6-inch round cake pan with olive oil cooking spray.
2. In a large bowl, beat the eggs for 1 to 2 minutes, or until well combined.
3. Add the bell pepper, salt, black pepper, and garlic to the eggs, and mix together until the bell pepper is distributed throughout.
4. Fold in ¼ cup of the feta cheese.
5. Pour the egg mixture into the prepared cake pan, and sprinkle the remaining ¼ cup of feta over the top.
6. Place into the air fryer and bake for 18 to 20 minutes, or until the eggs are set in the center.
7. Remove from the air fryer and allow to cool for 5 minutes before serving.

Per Serving
calories: 204 | fat: 14g | protein: 16g
carbs: 4g | fiber: 1g | sodium: 606mg

Shakshuka with Cilantro

Prep time: 15 minutes | Cook time: 18 minutes | Serves 4

2 tablespoons extra-virgin olive oil
1 cup chopped shallots
1 cup chopped red bell peppers
1 cup finely diced potato
1 teaspoon garlic powder
1 (14½-ounce / 411-g) can diced tomatoes, drained
¼ teaspoon turmeric
¼ teaspoon paprika
¼ teaspoon ground cardamom
4 large eggs
¼ cup chopped fresh cilantro

1. Preheat the oven to 350ºF (180ºC).
2. In an oven-safe sauté pan or skillet, heat the olive oil over medium-high heat and sauté the shallots, stirring occasionally, for about 3 minutes, until fragrant. Add the bell peppers, potato, and garlic powder. Cook, uncovered, for 10 minutes, stirring every 2 minutes.
3. Add the tomatoes, turmeric, paprika, and cardamom to the skillet and mix well. Once bubbly, remove from heat and crack the eggs into the skillet so the yolks are facing up.
4. Put the skillet in the oven and cook for an additional 5 to 10 minutes, until eggs are cooked to your preference. Garnish with the cilantro and serve.

Per Serving
calories: 224 | fat: 12g | protein: 9g
carbs: 20g | fiber: 3g | sodium: 278mg

Veggie Stuffed Hash Browns

Prep time: 10 minutes | Cook time: 20 minutes | Serves 4

Olive oil cooking spray
1 tablespoon plus 2 teaspoons olive oil, divided
4 ounces (113 g) baby bella mushrooms, diced
1 scallion, white parts and green parts, diced
1 garlic clove, minced
2 cups shredded potatoes
½ teaspoon salt
¼ teaspoon black pepper
1 Roma tomato, diced
½ cup shredded Mozzarella

1. Preheat the air fryer to 380ºF (193ºC). Lightly coat the inside of a 6-inch cake pan with olive oil cooking spray.
2. In a small skillet, heat 2 teaspoons olive oil over medium heat. Add the mushrooms, scallion, and garlic, and cook for 4 to 5 minutes, or until they have softened and are beginning to show some color. Remove from heat.
3. Meanwhile, in a large bowl, combine the potatoes, salt, pepper, and the remaining tablespoon olive oil. Toss until all potatoes are well coated.
4. Pour half of the potatoes into the bottom of the cake pan. Top with the mushroom mixture, tomato, and Mozzarella. Spread the remaining potatoes over the top.
5. Bake in the air fryer for 12 to 15 minutes, or until the top is golden brown.
6. Remove from the air fryer and allow to cool for 5 minutes before slicing and serving.

Per Serving
calories: 164 | fat: 9g | protein: 6g
carbs: 16g | fiber: 3g | sodium: 403mg

Healthy Green Smoothie

Prep time: 10 minutes | Cook time: 0 minutes | Serves 1

1 small very ripe avocado, peeled and pitted
1 cup almond milk or water, plus more as needed
1 cup tender baby spinach leaves, stems removed
½ medium cucumber, peeled and seeded
1 tablespoon extra-virgin olive oil or avocado oil
8 to 10 fresh mint leaves, stems removed
1 to 2 tablespoons juice of 1 lime

1. In a blender or a large wide-mouth jar, if using an immersion blender, combine the avocado, almond milk, spinach, cucumber, olive oil, mint, and lime juice and blend until smooth and creamy, adding more almond milk or water to achieve your desired consistency.

Per Serving
calories: 330 | fat: 30g | protein: 4g
carbs: 19g | fiber: 8g | sodium: 36mg

Vanilla Raspberry Overnight Oats
Prep time: 10 minutes | Cook time: 0 minutes | Serves 2

⅔ cup vanilla, unsweetened almond milk
⅓ cup rolled oats
¼ cup raspberries
1 teaspoon honey
¼ teaspoon turmeric
⅛ teaspoon ground cinnamon
Pinch ground cloves

1. In a mason jar, combine the almond milk, oats, raspberries, honey, turmeric, cinnamon, and cloves and shake well. Store in the refrigerator for 8 to 24 hours, then serve cold or heated.

Per Serving
calories: 82 | fat: 2g | protein: 2g
carbs: 14g | fiber: 3g | sodium: 98mg

Tomato, Herb, and Goat Cheese Frittata
Prep time: 15 minutes | Cook time: 25 minutes | Serves 2

1 tablespoon olive oil
½ pint cherry or grape tomatoes
2 garlic cloves, minced
5 large eggs, beaten
3 tablespoons unsweetened almond milk
½ teaspoon salt
Pinch freshly ground black pepper
2 tablespoons minced fresh oregano
2 tablespoons minced fresh basil
2 ounces (57 g) crumbled goat cheese (about ½ cup)

1. Heat the oil in a nonstick skillet over medium heat. Add the tomatoes. As they start to cook, pierce some of them so they give off some of their juice. Reduce the heat to medium-low, cover the pan, and let the tomatoes soften.
2. When the tomatoes are mostly softened and broken down, remove the lid, add the garlic and continue to sauté.
3. In a medium bowl, combine the eggs, milk, salt, pepper, and herbs and whisk well to combine.
4. Turn the heat up to medium-high. Add the egg mixture to the tomatoes and garlic, then sprinkle the goat cheese over the eggs.
5. Cover the pan and let cook for about 7 minutes.
6. Uncover the pan and continue cooking for another 7 to 10 minutes, or until the eggs are set. Run a spatula around the edge of the pan to make sure they won't stick.
7. Let the frittata cool for about 5 minutes before serving. Cut it into wedges and serve.

Per Serving
calories: 417 | fat: 31g | protein: 26g
carbs: 12g | fiber: 3g | sodium: 867mg

Pumpkin Muffins
Prep time: 15 minutes | Cook time: 15 minutes | Makes 12 muffins

Nonstick cooking spray
1½ cups granulated sugar
½ cup sugar
¾ cup all-purpose flour
2 teaspoons pumpkin pie spice
1 teaspoon baking soda
¼ teaspoon salt
Pinch nutmeg
3 mashed bananas
1 (15-ounce / 425-g) can pure pumpkin purée
½ cup plain, unsweetened, full-fat yogurt
½ cup butter, melted (optional)
2 large egg whites

1. Preheat the oven to 350ºF (180ºC). Spray a muffin tin with cooking spray.
2. In a large bowl, mix the sugars, flour, pumpkin pie spice, baking soda, salt, and nutmeg. In a separate bowl, mix the bananas, pumpkin purée, yogurt, and butter (if desired). Slowly mix the wet ingredients into the dry ingredients.
3. In a large glass bowl, using a mixer on high, whip the egg whites until stiff and fold them into the batter.
4. Pour the batter into a muffin tin, filling each cup halfway. Bake for 15 minutes, or until a fork inserted in the center comes out clean.

Per Serving
calories: 259 | fat: 8g | protein: 3g
carbs: 49g | fiber: 3g | sodium: 226mg

Avocado Smoothie

Prep time: 2 minutes | Cook time: 0 minutes | Serves 2

1 large avocado
1½ cups unsweetened coconut
milk
2 tablespoons honey

1. Place all ingredients in a blender and blend until smooth and creamy. Serve immediately.

Per Serving
calories: 686 | fat: 57g | protein: 6g
carbs: 35g | fiber: 10g | sodium: 35mg

Baked Ricotta with Honey Pears

Prep time: 5 minutes | Cook time: 22 to 25 minutes | Serves 4

1 (1-pound / 454-g) container whole-milk ricotta cheese
2 large eggs
¼ cup whole-wheat pastry flour
1 tablespoon sugar
1 teaspoon vanilla extract
¼ teaspoon ground nutmeg
1 pear, cored and diced
2 tablespoons water
1 tablespoon honey
Nonstick cooking spray

1. Preheat the oven to 400ºF (205ºC). Spray four ramekins with nonstick cooking spray.
2. Beat together the ricotta, eggs, flour, sugar, vanilla, and nutmeg in a large bowl until combined. Spoon the mixture into the ramekins.
3. Bake in the preheated oven for 22 to 25 minutes, or until the ricotta is just set.
4. Meanwhile, in a small saucepan over medium heat, simmer the pear in the water for 10 minutes, or until slightly softened. Remove from the heat, and stir in the honey.
5. Remove the ramekins from the oven and cool slightly on a wire rack. Top the ricotta ramekins with the pear and serve.

Per Serving
calories: 329 | fat: 19g | protein: 17g
carbs: 23g | fiber: 3g | sodium: 109mg

Feta and Olive Scrambled Eggs

Prep time: 5 minutes | Cook time: 5 minutes | Serves 2

4 large eggs
1 tablespoon unsweetened almond milk
Sea salt and freshly ground pepper, to taste
1 tablespoon olive oil
¼ cup crumbled feta cheese
10 Kalamata olives, pitted and sliced
Small bunch fresh mint, chopped, for garnish

1. Beat the eggs in a bowl until just combined. Add the milk and a pinch of sea salt and whisk well.
2. Heat a medium nonstick skillet over medium-high heat and add the olive oil.
3. Pour in the egg mixture and stir constantly, or until they just begin to curd and firm up, about 2 minutes. Add the feta cheese and olive slices, and stir until evenly combined. Season to taste with salt and pepper.
4. Divide the mixture between 2 plates and serve garnished with the fresh chopped mint.

Per Serving
calories: 244 | fat: 21g | protein: 8g
carbs: 3g | fiber: 0g | sodium: 339mg

Apple-Tahini Toast

Prep time: 5 minutes | Cook time: 0 minutes | Serves 1

2 slices whole-wheat bread, toasted
2 tablespoons tahini
1 small apple of your
choice, cored and thinly sliced
1 teaspoon honey

1. Spread the tahini on the toasted bread.
2. Place the apple slices on the bread and drizzle with the honey. Serve immediately.

Per Serving
calories: 458 | fat: 17g | protein: 11g
carbs: 63g | fiber: 10g | sodium: 285mg

Tuna and Avocado Salad Sandwich
Prep time: 10 minutes | Cook time: 2 minutes | Serves 4

- 4 versatile sandwich rounds
- 2 (4-ounce/ 113-g) cans tuna, packed in olive oil
- 2 tablespoons roasted garlic aioli, or avocado oil mayonnaise with 1 to
- 2 teaspoons freshly squeezed lemon juice
- and/or zest
- 1 very ripe avocado, peeled, pitted, and mashed
- 1 tablespoon chopped fresh capers (optional)
- 1 teaspoon chopped fresh dill or ½ teaspoon dried dill

1. Make sandwich rounds according to recipe. Cut each round in half and set aside.
2. In a medium bowl, place the tuna and the oil from cans. Add the aioli, avocado, capers (if using), and dill and blend well with a fork.
3. Toast sandwich rounds and fill each with one-quarter of the tuna salad, about ⅓ cup.

Per Serving (1 sandwich)
calories: 436 | fat: 36g | protein: 23g
carbs: 5g | fiber: 3g | sodium: 790mg

Breakfast Pancakes with Berry Sauce
Prep time: 5 minutes | Cook time: 10 minutes | Serves 4

Pancakes:
1 cup almond flour
1 teaspoon baking powder
¼ teaspoon salt
6 tablespoon extra-virgin olive oil,
divided
2 large eggs, beaten
Zest and juice of 1 lemon
½ teaspoon vanilla extract

Berry Sauce:
1 cup frozen mixed berries
1 tablespoon water,
plus more as needed
½ teaspoon vanilla extract

Make the Pancakes
1. In a large bowl, combine the almond flour, baking powder, and salt and stir to break up any clumps.

2. Add 4 tablespoons olive oil, beaten eggs, lemon zest and juice, and vanilla extract and stir until well mixed.
3. Heat 1 tablespoon of olive oil in a large skillet. Spoon about 2 tablespoons of batter for each pancake. Cook until bubbles begin to form, 4 to 5 minutes. Flip and cook for another 2 to 3 minutes. Repeat with the remaining 1 tablespoon of olive oil and batter.

Make the Berry Sauce
1. Combine the frozen berries, water, and vanilla extract in a small saucepan and heat over medium-high heat for 3 to 4 minutes until bubbly, adding more water as needed. Using the back of a spoon or fork, mash the berries and whisk until smooth.
2. Serve the pancakes with the berry sauce.

Per Serving
calories: 275 | fat: 26g | protein: 4g
carbs: 8g | fiber: 2g | sodium: 271mg

Fruity Pancakes with Berry-Honey Compote
Prep time: 10 minutes | Cook time: 4 minutes | Serves 4

1 cup almond flour
1 cup plus 2 tablespoons skim milk
2 large eggs, beaten
⅓ cup honey
1 teaspoon baking soda
¼ teaspoon salt
2 tablespoons extra-virgin olive oil
1 sliced banana or 1 cup sliced strawberries, divided
2 tablespoons berry and honey compote

1. In a bowl, mix together the almond flour, milk, eggs, honey, baking soda, and salt.
2. In a large sauté pan or skillet, heat the olive oil over medium-high heat and pour ⅓ cup pancake batter into the pan. Cook for 2 to 3 minutes. Right before pancake is ready to flip, add half of the fresh fruit and flip to cook for 2 to 3 minutes on the other side, until cooked through.
3. Top with the remaining fruit, drizzle with berry and honey compote and serve.

Per Serving
calories: 415 | fat: 24g | protein: 12| carbs: 46g | fiber: 4g | sodium: 526mg

Tangy Almond-Pistachio Smoothie

Prep time: 10 minutes | Cook time: 0 minutes | Serves 1

½ cup plain whole-milk Greek yogurt
½ cup unsweetened almond milk, plus more as needed
Zest and juice of 1 clementine or ½ orange
1 tablespoon extra-virgin olive oil or MCT oil
1 tablespoon shelled pistachios, coarsely chopped
1 to 2 teaspoons monk fruit extract or stevia (optional)
¼ to ½ teaspoon ground allspice or unsweetened pumpkin pie spice
¼ teaspoon ground cinnamon
¼ teaspoon vanilla extract

1. In a blender or a large wide-mouth jar, if using an immersion blender, combine the yogurt, ½ cup almond milk, clementine zest and juice, olive oil, pistachios, monk fruit extract (if using), allspice, cinnamon, and vanilla and blend until smooth and creamy, adding more almond milk to achieve your desired consistency.

Per Serving
calories: 264 | fat: 22g | protein: 5g
carbs: 12g | fiber: 1g | sodium: 127mg

Marinara Poached Eggs

Prep time: 5 minutes | Cook time: 15 minutes | Serves 6

1 tablespoon extra-virgin olive oil
1 cup chopped onion
2 garlic cloves, minced
2 (14.5-ounce / 411-g) cans no-salt-added Italian diced tomatoes, undrained
6 large eggs
½ cup chopped fresh flat-leaf parsley

1. Heat the olive oil in a large skillet over medium-high heat.
2. Add the onion and sauté for 5 minutes, stirring occasionally. Add the garlic and cook for 1 minute more.
3. Pour the tomatoes with their juices over the onion mixture and cook for 2 to 3 minutes until bubbling.
4. Reduce the heat to medium and use a large spoon to make six indentations in the tomato mixture. Crack the eggs, one at a time, into each indentation.
5. Cover and simmer for 6 to 7 minutes, or until the eggs are cooked to your preference.
6. Serve with the parsley sprinkled on top.

Per Serving
calories: 89 | fat: 6g | protein: 4g
carbs: 4g | fiber: 1g | sodium: 77mg

Warm Bulgur Breakfast Bowls with Fruits

Prep time: 5 minutes | Cook time: 15 minutes | Serves 6

2 cups unsweetened almond milk
1½ cups uncooked bulgur
1 cup water
½ teaspoon ground cinnamon
2 cups frozen (or fresh, pitted) dark sweet cherries
8 dried (or fresh) figs, chopped
½ cup chopped almonds
¼ cup loosely packed fresh mint, chopped

1. Combine the milk, bulgur, water, and cinnamon in a medium saucepan, stirring, and bring just to a boil.
2. Cover, reduce the heat to medium-low, and allow to simmer for 10 minutes, or until the liquid is absorbed.
3. Turn off the heat, but keep the pan on the stove, and stir in the frozen cherries (no need to thaw), figs, and almonds. Cover and let the hot bulgur thaw the cherries and partially hydrate the figs, about 1 minute.
4. Fold in the mint and stir to combine, then serve.

Per Serving
calories: 207 | fat: 6g | protein: 8g
carbs: 32g | fiber: 4g | sodium: 82mg

Mediterranean Herb Frittata

Prep time: 10 minutes | Cook time: 7 minutes | Serves 2

4 large eggs
2 tablespoons fresh chopped herbs, such as rosemary, thyme, oregano, basil or 1 teaspoon dried herbs
¼ teaspoon salt
Freshly ground black pepper, to taste
4 tablespoons extra-virgin olive oil, divided

1 cup fresh spinach, arugula, kale, or other leafy greens
4 ounces (113 g) quartered artichoke hearts, rinsed, drained, and thoroughly dried
8 cherry tomatoes, halved
½ cup crumbled soft goat cheese

1. Preheat the oven to broil on low.
2. In small bowl, combine the eggs, herbs, salt, and pepper and whisk well with a fork. Set aside.
3. In a 4- to 5-inch oven-safe skillet or omelet pan, heat 2 tablespoons olive oil over medium heat. Add the spinach, artichoke hearts, and cherry tomatoes and sauté until just wilted, 1 to 2 minutes.
4. Pour in the egg mixture and let it cook undisturbed over medium heat for 3 to 4 minutes, until the eggs begin to set on the bottom.
5. Sprinkle the goat cheese across the top of the egg mixture and transfer the skillet to the oven.
6. Broil for 4 to 5 minutes, or until the frittata is firm in the center and golden brown on top.
7. Remove from the oven and run a rubber spatula around the edge to loosen the sides. Invert onto a large plate or cutting board and slice in half. Serve warm and drizzled with the remaining 2 tablespoons olive oil.

Per Serving
calories: 527 | fat: 47g | protein: 21g
carbs: 10g | fiber: 3g | sodium: 760mg

Hearty Honey-Apricot Granola

Prep time: 15 minutes | Cook time: 30 minutes | Serves 6

1 cup rolled oats
¼ cup dried apricots, diced
¼ cup almond slivers
¼ cup walnuts, chopped
¼ cup pumpkin seeds
¼ cup hemp hearts
¼ to ⅓ cup raw honey, plus more for drizzling

1 tablespoon olive oil
1 teaspoon ground cinnamon
¼ teaspoon ground nutmeg
¼ teaspoon salt
2 tablespoons sugar-free dark chocolate chips (optional)
3 cups nonfat plain Greek yogurt

1. Preheat the air fryer to 260ºF (127ºC). Line the air fryer basket with parchment paper.
2. In a large bowl, combine the oats, apricots, almonds, walnuts, pumpkin seeds, hemp hearts, honey, olive oil, cinnamon, nutmeg, and salt, mixing so that the honey, oil, and spices are well distributed.
3. Pour the mixture onto the parchment paper and spread it into an even layer.
4. Bake for 10 minutes, then shake or stir and spread back out into an even layer. Continue baking for 10 minutes more, then repeat the process of shaking or stirring the mixture. Bake for an additional 10 minutes before removing from the air fryer.
5. Allow the granola to cool completely before stirring in the chocolate chips (if using) and pouring into an airtight container for storage.
6. For each serving, top ½ cup Greek yogurt with ⅓ cup granola and a drizzle of honey, if needed.

Per Serving
calories: 342 | fat: 16g | protein: 20g
carbs: 31g | fiber: 4g | sodium: 162mg

Polenta with Arugula, Figs, and Blue Cheese

Prep time: 10 minutes | Cook time: 40 minutes | Serves 4

1 cup coarse-ground cornmeal
½ cup oil-packed sun-dried tomatoes, chopped
1 teaspoon minced fresh thyme or ¼ teaspoon dried
½ teaspoon table salt
¼ teaspoon pepper
3 tablespoons extra-virgin olive oil,
divided
2 ounces (57 g) baby arugula
4 figs, cut into ½-inch-thick wedges
1 tablespoon balsamic vinegar
2 ounces (57 g) blue cheese, crumbled
2 tablespoons pine nuts, toasted

1. Arrange trivet included with Instant Pot in base of insert and add 1 cup water. Fold sheet of aluminum foil into 16 by 6-inch sling, then rest 1½-quart round soufflé dish in center of sling. Whisk 4 cups water, cornmeal, tomatoes, thyme, salt, and pepper together in bowl, then transfer mixture to soufflé dish. Using sling, lower soufflé dish into pot and onto trivet; allow narrow edges of sling to rest along sides of insert.
2. Lock lid in place and close pressure release valve. Select high pressure cook function and cook for 40 minutes. Turn off Instant Pot and quick-release pressure. Carefully remove lid, allowing steam to escape away from you.
3. Using sling, transfer soufflé dish to wire rack. Whisk 1 tablespoon oil into polenta, smoothing out any lumps. Let sit until thickened slightly, about 10 minutes. Season with salt and pepper to taste.
4. Toss arugula and figs with vinegar and remaining 2 tablespoons oil in bowl, and season with salt and pepper to taste. Divide polenta among individual serving plates and top with arugula mixture, blue cheese, and pine nuts. Serve.

Per Serving
calories: 360 | fat: 21g | protein: 7g
carbs: 38g | fiber: 8g | sodium: 510mg

Parmesan Spinach Pie

Prep time: 10 minutes | Cook time: 20 minutes | Serves 8

Nonstick cooking spray
2 tablespoons extra-virgin olive oil
1 onion, chopped
1 pound (454 g) frozen spinach, thawed
¼ teaspoon garlic salt
¼ teaspoon freshly ground black pepper
¼ teaspoon ground nutmeg
4 large eggs, divided
1 cup grated Parmesan cheese, divided
2 puff pastry doughs, (organic, if available), at room temperature
4 hard-boiled eggs, halved

1. Preheat the oven to 350ºF (180ºC). Spray a baking sheet with nonstick cooking spray and set aside.
2. Heat a large sauté pan or skillet over medium-high heat. Put in the oil and onion and cook for about 5 minutes, until translucent.
3. Squeeze the excess water from the spinach, then add to the pan and cook, uncovered, so that any excess water from the spinach can evaporate. Add the garlic salt, pepper, and nutmeg. Remove from heat and set aside to cool.
4. In a small bowl, crack 3 eggs and mix well. Add the eggs and ½ cup Parmesan cheese to the cooled spinach mix.
5. On the prepared baking sheet, roll out the pastry dough. Layer the spinach mix on top of dough, leaving 2 inches around each edge.
6. Once the spinach is spread onto the pastry dough, place hard-boiled egg halves evenly throughout the pie, then cover with the second pastry dough. Pinch the edges closed.
7. Crack the remaining egg in a small bowl and mix well. Brush the egg wash over the pastry dough.
8. Bake for 15 to 20 minutes, until golden brown and warmed through.

Per Serving
calories: 417 | fat: 28g | protein: 17g
carbs: 25g | fiber: 3g | sodium: 490mg

Prosciutto Breakfast Bruschetta

Prep time: 10 minutes | Cook time: 20 minutes | Serves 4

¼ teaspoon kosher or sea salt
6 cups broccoli rabe, stemmed and chopped (about 1 bunch)
1 tablespoon extra-virgin olive oil
2 garlic cloves, minced (about 1 teaspoon)
1 ounce (28 g) prosciutto, cut or torn into ½-inch pieces
¼ teaspoon crushed red pepper
Nonstick cooking spray
3 large eggs
1 tablespoon unsweetened almond milk
¼ teaspoon freshly ground black pepper
4 teaspoons grated Parmesan or Pecorino Romano cheese
1 garlic clove, halved
8 (¾-inch-thick) slices baguette-style whole-grain bread or 4 slices larger Italian-style whole-grain bread

1. Bring a large stockpot of water to a boil. Add the salt and broccoli rabe, and boil for 2 minutes. Drain in a colander.
2. In a large skillet over medium heat, heat the oil. Add the garlic, prosciutto, and crushed red pepper, and cook for 2 minutes, stirring often. Add the broccoli rabe and cook for an additional 3 minutes, stirring a few times. Transfer to a bowl and set aside.
3. Place the skillet back on the stove over low heat and coat with nonstick cooking spray.
4. In a small bowl, whisk together the eggs, milk, and pepper. Pour into the skillet. Stir and cook until the eggs are soft scrambled, 3 to 5 minutes. Add the broccoli rabe mixture back to the skillet along with the cheese. Stir and cook for about 1 minute, until heated through. Remove from the heat.
5. Toast the bread, then rub the cut sides of the garlic clove halves onto one side of each slice of the toast. (Save the garlic for another recipe.) Spoon the egg mixture onto each piece of toast and serve.

Per Serving
calories: 313 | fat: 10g | protein: 17g
carbs: 38g | fiber: 8g | sodium: 559mg

Chickpea and Hummus Patties in Pitas

Prep time: 15 minutes | Cook time: 13 minutes | Serves 4

1 (15-ounce / 425-g) can chickpeas, drained and rinsed
½ cup lemony garlic hummus or ½ cup prepared hummus
½ cup whole-wheat panko bread crumbs
1 large egg
2 teaspoons dried oregano
¼ teaspoon freshly ground black pepper
1 tablespoon extra-virgin olive oil
1 cucumber, unpeeled (or peeled if desired), cut in half lengthwise
1 (6-ounce / 170-g) container 2% plain Greek yogurt
1 garlic clove, minced
2 whole-wheat pita breads, cut in half
1 medium tomato, cut into 4 thick slices

1. In a large bowl, mash the chickpeas with a potato masher or fork until coarsely smashed (they should still be somewhat chunky). Add the hummus, bread crumbs, egg, oregano, and pepper. Stir well to combine. With your hands, form the mixture into 4 (½-cup-size) patties. Press each patty flat to about ¾ inch thick and put on a plate.
2. In a large skillet over medium-high heat, heat the oil until very hot, about 3 minutes. Cook the patties for 5 minutes, then flip with a spatula. Cook for an additional 5 minutes.
3. While the patties are cooking, shred half of the cucumber with a box grater or finely chop with a knife. In a small bowl, stir together the shredded cucumber, yogurt, and garlic to make the tzatziki sauce. Slice the remaining half of the cucumber into ¼-inch-thick slices and set aside.
4. Toast the pita breads. To assemble the sandwiches, lay the pita halves on a work surface. Into each pita, place a few slices of cucumber, a chickpea patty, and a tomato slice, then drizzle the sandwich with the tzatziki sauce and serve.

Per Serving
calories: 308 | fat: 8g | protein: 15g
carbs: 45g | fiber: 78g | sodium: 321mg

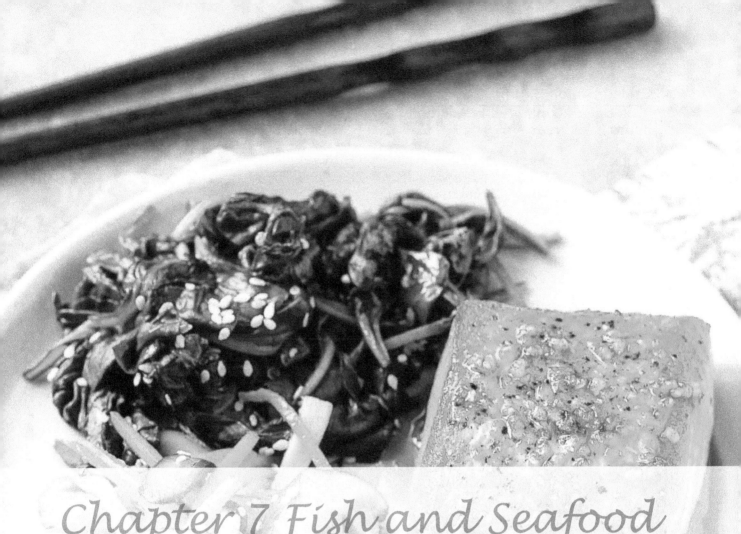
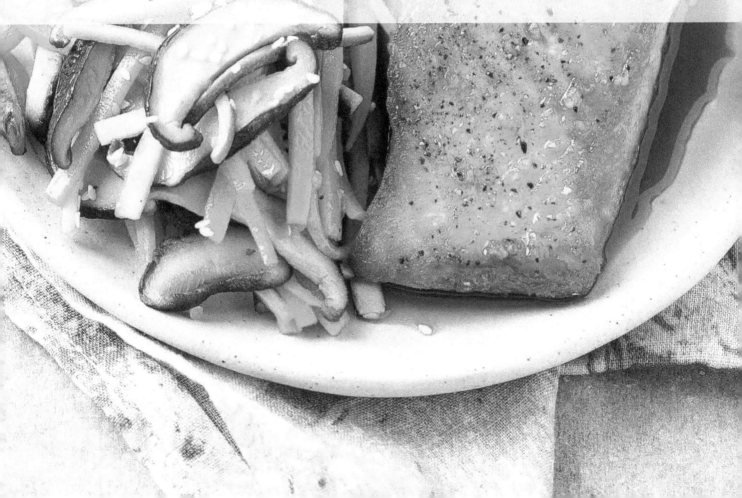

Chapter 7 Fish and Seafood

Grilled Lemon Shrimp

Prep time: 20 minutes | Cook time: 5 minutes | Serves 4 to 6

2 tablespoons garlic, minced
½ cup lemon juice
3 tablespoons fresh Italian parsley, finely chopped
¼ cup extra-virgin

olive oil
1 teaspoon salt
2 pounds (907 g) jumbo shrimp (21 to 25), peeled and deveined

1. In a large bowl, mix the garlic, lemon juice, parsley, olive oil, and salt.
2. Add the shrimp to the bowl and toss to make sure all the pieces are coated with the marinade. Let the shrimp sit for 15 minutes.
3. Preheat a grill, grill pan, or lightly oiled skillet to high heat. While heating, thread about 5 to 6 pieces of shrimp onto each skewer.
4. Place the skewers on the grill, grill pan, or skillet and cook for 2 to 3 minutes on each side until cooked through. Serve warm.

Per Serving
calories: 402 | fat: 18g | protein: 57g
carbs: 4g | fiber: 0g | sodium: 1224mg

Italian Fried Shrimp

Prep time: 10 minutes | Cook time: 5 minutes | Serves 4

2 large eggs
2 cups seasoned Italian bread crumbs
1 teaspoon salt
1 cup flour

1 pound (454 g) large shrimp (21 to 25), peeled and deveined
Extra-virgin olive oil

1. In a small bowl, beat the eggs with 1 tablespoon water, then transfer to a shallow dish.
2. Add the bread crumbs and salt to a separate shallow dish; mix well.
3. Place the flour into a third shallow dish.
4. Coat the shrimp in the flour, then egg, and finally the bread crumbs. Place on a plate and repeat with all of the shrimp.

5. Preheat a skillet over high heat. Pour in enough olive oil to coat the bottom of the skillet. Cook the shrimp in the hot skillet for 2 to 3 minutes on each side. Take the shrimp out and drain on a paper towel. Serve warm.

Per Serving
calories: 714 | fat: 34g | protein: 37g
carbs: 63g | fiber: 3g | sodium: 1727mg

Cod Saffron Rice

Prep time: 10 minutes | Cook time: 35 minutes | Serves 4

4 tablespoons extra-virgin olive oil, divided
1 large onion, chopped
3 cod fillets, rinsed and patted dry

4½ cups water
1 teaspoon saffron threads
1½ teaspoons salt
1 teaspoon turmeric
2 cups long-grain rice, rinsed

1. In a large pot over medium heat, cook 2 tablespoons of olive oil and the onions for 5 minutes.
2. While the onions are cooking, preheat another large pan over high heat. Add the remaining 2 tablespoons of olive oil and the cod fillets. Cook the cod for 2 minutes on each side, then remove from the pan and set aside.
3. Once the onions are done cooking, add the water, saffron, salt, turmeric, and rice, stirring to combine. Cover and cook for 12 minutes.
4. Cut the cod up into 1-inch pieces. Place the cod pieces in the rice, lightly toss, cover, and cook for another 10 minutes.
5. Once the rice is done cooking, fluff with a fork, cover, and let stand for 5 minutes. Serve warm.

Per Serving
calories: 564 | fat: 15g | protein: 26g
carbs: 78g | fiber: 2g | sodium: 945mg

Easy Tuna Steaks

Prep time: 10 minutes | Cook time: 8 minutes | Serves 4

1 teaspoon garlic powder
½ teaspoon salt
¼ teaspoon dried thyme
¼ teaspoon dried oregano
4 tuna steaks
2 tablespoons olive oil
1 lemon, quartered

1. Preheat the air fryer to 380ºF (193ºC).
2. In a small bowl, whisk together the garlic powder, salt, thyme, and oregano.
3. Coat the tuna steaks with olive oil. Season both sides of each steak with the seasoning blend. Place the steaks in a single layer in the air fryer basket.
4. Cook for 5 minutes, then flip and cook for an additional 3 to 4 minutes.

Per Serving
calories: 269 | fat: 13g | protein: 33g
carbs: 1g | fiber: 0g | sodium: 231mg

Honey-Garlic Glazed Salmon

Prep time: 5 minutes | Cook time: 10 minutes | Serves 4

¼ cup raw honey
4 garlic cloves, minced
1 tablespoon olive oil
½ teaspoon salt
Olive oil cooking spray
4 (1½-inch-thick) salmon fillets

1. Preheat the air fryer to 380ºF (193ºC).
2. In a small bowl, mix together the honey, garlic, olive oil, and salt.
3. Spray the bottom of the air fryer basket with olive oil cooking spray, and place the salmon in a single layer on the bottom of the air fryer basket.
4. Brush the top of each fillet with the honey-garlic mixture, and roast for 10 to 12 minutes, or until the internal temperature reaches 145ºF (63ºC).

Per Serving
calories: 260 | fat: 10g | protein: 23g
carbs: 18g | fiber: 0g | sodium: 342mg

Balsamic Shrimp on Tomato and Olive

Prep time: 10 minutes | Cook time: 6 minutes | Serves 4

½ cup olive oil
4 garlic cloves, minced
1 tablespoon balsamic vinegar
¼ teaspoon cayenne pepper
¼ teaspoon salt
1 Roma tomato, diced
¼ cup Kalamata olives
1 pound (454 g) medium shrimp, cleaned and deveined

1. Preheat the air fryer to 380ºF (193ºC).
2. In a small bowl, combine the olive oil, garlic, balsamic, cayenne, and salt.
3. Divide the tomatoes and olives among four small ramekins. Then divide shrimp among the ramekins, and pour a quarter of the oil mixture over the shrimp.
4. Cook for 6 to 8 minutes, or until the shrimp are cooked through.

Per Serving
calories: 160 | fat: 8g | protein: 16g
carbs: 4g | fiber: 1g | sodium: 213mg

Grouper Fillet with Tomato and Olive

Prep time: 10 minutes | Cook time: 10 minutes | Serves 4

4 grouper fillets
½ teaspoon salt
3 garlic cloves, minced
1 tomato, sliced
¼ cup sliced
Kalamata olives
¼ cup fresh dill, roughly chopped
Juice of 1 lemon
¼ cup olive oil

1. Preheat the air fryer to 380ºF (193ºC).
2. Season the grouper fillets on all sides with salt, then place into the air fryer basket and top with the minced garlic, tomato slices, olives, and fresh dill.
3. Drizzle the lemon juice and olive oil over the top of the grouper, then bake for 10 to 12 minutes, or until the internal temperature reaches 145ºF (63ºC),

Per Serving
calories: 271 | fat: 15g | protein: 28g
carbs: 3g | fiber: 1g | sodium: 324mg

Thyme Whole Roasted Red Snapper

Prep time: 5 minutes | Cook time: 45 minutes | Serves 4

1 (2 to 2½ pounds / 907 g to 1.1 kg) whole red snapper, cleaned and scaled
2 lemons, sliced (about 10 slices)
3 cloves garlic, sliced

4 or 5 sprigs of thyme
3 tablespoons cold salted butter, cut into small cubes, divided (optional)

1. Preheat the oven to 350ºF (180ºC).
2. Cut a piece of foil to about the size of your baking sheet; put the foil on the baking sheet.
3. Make a horizontal slice through the belly of the fish to create a pocket.
4. Place 3 slices of lemon on the foil and the fish on top of the lemons.
5. Stuff the fish with the garlic, thyme, 3 lemon slices and butter. Reserve 3 pieces of butter.
6. Place the reserved 3 pieces of butter on top of the fish, and 3 or 4 slices of lemon on top of the butter. Bring the foil together and seal it to make a pocket around the fish.
7. Put the fish in the oven and bake for 45 minutes. Serve with remaining fresh lemon slices.

Per Serving
calories: 345 | fat: 13g | protein: 54g
carbs: 12g | fiber: 3g | sodium: 170mg

Crispy Fried Sardines

Prep time: 5 minutes | Cook time: 5 minutes | Serves 4

Avocado oil, as needed
1½ pounds (680 g) whole fresh sardines, scales removed

1 teaspoon salt
1 teaspoon freshly ground black pepper
2 cups flour

1. Preheat a deep skillet over medium heat. Pour in enough oil so there is about 1 inch of it in the pan.
2. Season the fish with the salt and pepper.
3. Dredge the fish in the flour so it is completely covered.
4. Slowly drop in 1 fish at a time, making sure not to overcrowd the pan.

5. Cook for about 3 minutes on each side or just until the fish begins to brown on all sides. Serve warm.

Per Serving
calories: 794 | fat: 47g | protein: 48g
carbs: 44g | fiber: 2g | sodium: 1441mg

Fideos with Seafood

Prep time: 15 minutes | Cook time: 20 minutes | Serves 6 to 8

2 tablespoons extra-virgin olive oil, plus ½ cup, divided
6 cups zucchini noodles, roughly chopped (2 to 3 medium zucchini)
1 pound (454 g) shrimp, peeled, deveined and roughly chopped
6 to 8 ounces (170 to 227 g) canned chopped clams, drained
4 ounces (113 g) crab meat
½ cup crumbled goat

cheese
½ cup crumbled feta cheese
1 (28-ounce / 794-g) can chopped tomatoes, with their juices
1 teaspoon salt
1 teaspoon garlic powder
½ teaspoon smoked paprika
½ cup shredded Parmesan cheese
¼ cup chopped fresh flat-leaf Italian parsley, for garnish

1. Preheat the oven to 375ºF (190ºC).
2. Pour 2 tablespoons olive oil in the bottom of a 9-by-13-inch baking dish and swirl to coat the bottom.
3. In a large bowl, combine the zucchini noodles, shrimp, clams, and crab meat.
4. In another bowl, combine the goat cheese, feta, and ¼ cup olive oil and stir to combine well. Add the canned tomatoes and their juices, salt, garlic powder, and paprika and combine well. Add the mixture to the zucchini and seafood mixture and stir to combine.
5. Pour the mixture into the prepared baking dish, spreading evenly. Spread shredded Parmesan over top and drizzle with the remaining ¼ cup olive oil. Bake until bubbly, 20 to 25 minutes. Serve warm, garnished with chopped parsley.

Per Serving
calories: 434 | fat: 31g | protein: 29g
carbs: 12g | fiber: 3g | sodium: 712mg

Shrimp with Garlic and Mushrooms

Prep time: 10 minutes | Cook time: 15 minutes | Serves 4

1 pound (454 g) peeled and deveined fresh shrimp
1 teaspoon salt
1 cup extra-virgin olive oil
8 large garlic cloves, thinly sliced
4 ounces (113 g) sliced mushrooms
(shiitake, baby bella, or button)
½ teaspoon red pepper flakes
¼ cup chopped fresh flat-leaf Italian parsley
Zucchini noodles or riced cauliflower, for serving

1. Rinse the shrimp and pat dry. Place in a small bowl and sprinkle with the salt.
2. In a large rimmed, thick skillet, heat the olive oil over medium-low heat. Add the garlic and heat until very fragrant, 3 to 4 minutes, reducing the heat if the garlic starts to burn.
3. Add the mushrooms and sauté for 5 minutes, until softened. Add the shrimp and red pepper flakes and sauté until the shrimp begins to turn pink, another 3 to 4 minutes.
4. Remove from the heat and stir in the parsley. Serve over zucchini noodles or riced cauliflower.

Per Serving
calories: 620 | fat: 56g | protein: 24g
carbs: 4g | fiber: 0g | sodium: 736mg

Seafood Risotto

Prep time: 10 minutes | Cook time: 30 minutes | Serves 4

6 cups vegetable broth
3 tablespoons extra-virgin olive oil
1 large onion, chopped
3 cloves garlic, minced
½ teaspoon saffron
threads
1½ cups arborio rice
1½ teaspoons salt
8 ounces (227 g) shrimp (21 to 25), peeled and deveined
8 ounces (227 g) scallops

1. In a large saucepan over medium heat, bring the broth to a low simmer.
2. In a large skillet over medium heat, cook the olive oil, onion, garlic, and saffron for 3 minutes.
3. Add the rice, salt, and 1 cup of the broth to the skillet. Stir the ingredients together and cook over low heat until most of the liquid is absorbed. Repeat steps with broth, adding ½ cup of broth at a time, and cook until all but ½ cup of the broth is absorbed.
4. Add the shrimp and scallops when you stir in the final ½ cup of broth. Cover and let cook for 10 minutes. Serve warm.

Per Serving
calories: 460 | fat: 12g | protein: 24g
carbs: 64g | fiber: 2g | sodium: 2432mg

Dill and Garlic Stuffed Red Snapper

Prep time: 10 minutes | Cook time: 35 minutes | Serves 4

1 teaspoon salt
½ teaspoon black pepper
½ teaspoon ground cumin
¼ teaspoon cayenne
1 (1- to 1½-pound / 454- to 680-g) whole red snapper, cleaned
and patted dry
2 tablespoons olive oil
2 garlic cloves, minced
¼ cup fresh dill
Lemon wedges, for serving

1. Preheat the air fryer to 360ºF (182ºC)
2. In a small bowl, mix together the salt, pepper, cumin, and cayenne.
3. Coat the outside of the fish with olive oil, then sprinkle the seasoning blend over the outside of the fish. Stuff the minced garlic and dill inside the cavity of the fish.
4. Place the snapper into the basket of the air fryer and roast for 20 minutes. Flip the snapper over, and roast for 15 minutes more, or until the snapper reaches an internal temperature of 145ºF (63ºC).

Per Serving
calories: 125 | fat: 1g | protein: 23g
carbs: 2g | fiber: 0g | sodium: 562mg

Pollock and Vegetable Pitas

Prep time: 10 minutes | Cook time: 15 minutes | Serves 4

1 pound (454 g) pollock, cut into 1-inch pieces
¼ cup olive oil
1 teaspoon salt
½ teaspoon dried oregano
½ teaspoon dried thyme
½ teaspoon garlic powder
¼ teaspoon cayenne
4 whole wheat pitas
1 cup shredded lettuce
2 Roma tomatoes, diced
Nonfat plain Greek yogurt
Lemon, quartered

1. Preheat the air fryer to 380ºF (193ºC).
2. In a medium bowl, combine the pollock with olive oil, salt, oregano, thyme, garlic powder, and cayenne.
3. Put the pollock into the air fryer basket and cook for 15 minutes.
4. Serve inside pitas with lettuce, tomato, and Greek yogurt with a lemon wedge on the side.

Per Serving
calories: 368 | fat: 1g | protein: 21g
carbs: 38g | fiber: 5g | sodium: 514mg

Classic Escabeche

Prep time: 10 minutes | Cook time: 20 minutes | Serves 4

1 pound (454 g) wild-caught Spanish mackerel fillets, cut into four pieces
1 teaspoon salt
½ teaspoon freshly ground black pepper
8 tablespoons extra-virgin olive oil, divided
1 bunch asparagus, trimmed and cut into 2-inch pieces
1 (13¾-ounce / 390-g) can artichoke hearts, drained and quartered
4 large garlic cloves, peeled and crushed
2 bay leaves
¼ cup red wine vinegar
½ teaspoon smoked paprika

1. Sprinkle the fillets with salt and pepper and let sit at room temperature for 5 minutes.
2. In a large skillet, heat 2 tablespoons olive oil over medium-high heat. Add the fish, skin-side up, and cook 5 minutes.

Flip and cook 5 minutes on the other side, until browned and cooked through. Transfer to a serving dish, pour the cooking oil over the fish, and cover to keep warm.
3. Heat the remaining 6 tablespoons olive oil in the same skillet over medium heat. Add the asparagus, artichokes, garlic, and bay leaves and sauté until the vegetables are tender, 6 to 8 minutes.
4. Using a slotted spoon, top the fish with the cooked vegetables, reserving the oil in the skillet. Add the vinegar and paprika to the oil and whisk to combine well. Pour the vinaigrette over the fish and vegetables and let sit at room temperature for at least 15 minutes, or marinate in the refrigerator up to 24 hours for a deeper flavor. Remove the bay leaf before serving.

Per Serving
calories: 578 | fat: 50g | protein: 26g
carbs: 13g | fiber: 5g | sodium: 946mg

Cilantro Lemon Shrimp

Prep time: 20 minutes | Cook time: 10 minutes | Serves 4

⅓ cup lemon juice
4 garlic cloves
1 cup fresh cilantro leaves
½ teaspoon ground coriander
3 tablespoons extra-virgin olive oil
1 teaspoon salt
1½ pounds (680 g) large shrimp (21 to 25), deveined and shells removed

1. In a food processor, pulse the lemon juice, garlic, cilantro, coriander, olive oil, and salt 10 times.
2. Put the shrimp in a bowl or plastic zip-top bag, pour in the cilantro marinade, and let sit for 15 minutes.
3. Preheat a skillet on high heat.
4. Put the shrimp and marinade in the skillet. Cook the shrimp for 3 minutes on each side. Serve warm.

Per Serving
calories: 225 | fat: 12g | protein: 28g
carbs: 5g | fiber: 1g | sodium: 763mg

Fast Seafood Paella

Prep time: 20 minutes | Cook time: 20 minutes | Serves 4

¼ cup plus 1 tablespoon extra-virgin olive oil
1 large onion, finely chopped
2 tomatoes, peeled and chopped
1½ tablespoons garlic powder
1½ cups medium-grain Spanish paella rice or arborio rice
2 carrots, finely diced
Salt, to taste
1 tablespoon sweet paprika
8 ounces (227 g) lobster meat or canned crab
½ cup frozen peas
3 cups chicken stock, plus more if needed
1 cup dry white wine
6 jumbo shrimp, unpeeled
⅓ pound (136 g) calamari rings
1 lemon, halved

1. In a large sauté pan or skillet (16-inch is ideal), heat the oil over medium heat until small bubbles start to escape from oil. Add the onion and cook for about 3 minutes, until fragrant, then add tomatoes and garlic powder. Cook for 5 to 10 minutes, until the tomatoes are reduced by half and the consistency is sticky.
2. Stir in the rice, carrots, salt, paprika, lobster, and peas and mix well. In a pot or microwave-safe bowl, heat the chicken stock to almost boiling, then add it to the rice mixture. Bring to a simmer, then add the wine.
3. Smooth out the rice in the bottom of the pan. Cover and cook on low for 10 minutes, mixing occasionally, to prevent burning.
4. Top the rice with the shrimp, cover, and cook for 5 more minutes. Add additional broth to the pan if the rice looks dried out.
5. Right before removing the skillet from the heat, add the calamari rings. Toss the ingredients frequently. In about 2 minutes, the rings will look opaque. Remove the pan from the heat immediately (if you don't want the paella to overcook). Squeeze fresh lemon juice over the dish.

Per Serving
calories: 632 | fat: 20g | protein: 34g
carbs: 71g | fiber: 5g | sodium: 920mg

Lemon Rosemary Branzino

Prep time: 15 minutes | Cook time: 30 minutes | Serves 2

4 tablespoons extra-virgin olive oil, divided
2 (8-ounce / 227-g) branzino fillets, preferably at least 1 inch thick
1 garlic clove, minced
1 bunch scallions, white part only, thinly sliced
½ cup sliced pitted Kalamata or other good-quality black olives
1 large carrot, cut into ¼-inch rounds
10 to 12 small cherry tomatoes, halved
½ cup dry white wine
2 tablespoons paprika
2 teaspoons kosher salt
½ tablespoon ground chili pepper, preferably Turkish or Aleppo
2 rosemary sprigs or 1 tablespoon dried rosemary
1 small lemon, very thinly sliced

1. Warm a large, oven-safe sauté pan or skillet over high heat until hot, about 2 minutes. Carefully add 1 tablespoon of olive oil and heat until it shimmers, 10 to 15 seconds. Brown the branzino fillets for 2 minutes, skin-side up. Carefully flip the fillets skin-side down and cook for another 2 minutes, until browned. Set aside.
2. Swirl 2 tablespoons of olive oil around the skillet to coat evenly. Add the garlic, scallions, kalamata olives, carrot, and tomatoes, and let the vegetables sauté for 5 minutes, until softened. Add the wine, stirring until all ingredients are well integrated. Carefully place the fish over the sauce.
3. Preheat the oven to 450ºF (235ºC).
4. While the oven is heating, brush the fillets with 1 tablespoon of olive oil and season with paprika, salt, and chili pepper. Top each fillet with a rosemary sprig and several slices of lemon. Scatter the olives over fish and around the pan.
5. Roast until lemon slices are browned or singed, about 10 minutes.

Per Serving
calories: 725 | fat: 43g | protein: 58g
carbs: 25g | fiber: 10g | sodium: 2954mg

Orange Roasted Salmon

Prep time: 10 minutes | Cook time: 25 minutes | Serves 4

½ cup extra-virgin olive oil, divided
2 tablespoons balsamic vinegar
2 tablespoons garlic powder, divided
1 tablespoon cumin seeds
1 teaspoon sea salt, divided
1 teaspoon freshly ground black pepper, divided
2 teaspoons smoked paprika
4 (8-ounce / 227-g) salmon fillets, skinless
2 small red onion, thinly sliced
½ cup halved

Campari tomatoes
1 small fennel bulb, thinly sliced lengthwise
1 large carrot, thinly sliced
8 medium portobello mushrooms
8 medium radishes, sliced ⅛ inch thick
½ cup dry white wine
½ lime, zested
Handful cilantro leaves
½ cup halved pitted Kalamata olives
1 orange, thinly sliced
4 roasted sweet potatoes, cut in wedges lengthwise

1. Preheat the oven to 375ºF (190ºC).
2. In a medium bowl, mix 6 tablespoons of olive oil, the balsamic vinegar, 1 tablespoon of garlic powder, the cumin seeds, ¼ teaspoon of sea salt, ¼ teaspoon of pepper, and the paprika. Put the salmon in the bowl and marinate while preparing the vegetables, about 10 minutes.
3. Heat an oven-safe sauté pan or skillet on medium-high heat and sear the top of the salmon for about 2 minutes, or until lightly brown. Set aside.
4. Add the remaining 2 tablespoons of olive oil to the same skillet. Once it's hot, add the onion, tomatoes, fennel, carrot, mushrooms, radishes, the remaining 1 teaspoon of garlic powder, ¾ teaspoon of salt, and ¾ teaspoon of pepper. Mix well and cook for 5 to 7 minutes, until fragrant. Add wine and mix well.
5. Place the salmon on top of the vegetable mixture, browned-side up. Sprinkle the fish with lime zest and cilantro and place the olives around the fish. Put orange slices over the fish and cook for about 7 additional minutes. While this is baking, add the sliced sweet potato wedges on a baking sheet and bake this alongside the skillet.
6. Remove from the oven, cover the skillet tightly, and let rest for about 3 minutes.

Per Serving
calories: 841 | fat: 41g | protein: 59g
carbs: 60g | fiber: 15g | sodium: 908mg

Panko-Crusted Fish Sticks

Prep time: 10 minutes | Cook time: 5 minutes | Serves 4

2 large eggs, lightly beaten 1 tablespoon 2% milk
1 pound (454 g) skinned fish fillets (cod, tilapia, or other white fish) about ½ inch thick, sliced into 20 (1-inch-wide) strips
½ cup yellow cornmeal

½ cup whole-wheat panko bread crumbs or whole-wheat bread crumbs
¼ teaspoon smoked paprika
¼ teaspoon kosher or sea salt
¼ teaspoon freshly ground black pepper
Nonstick cooking spray

1. Place a large, rimmed baking sheet in the oven. Preheat the oven to 400ºF (205ºC) with the pan inside.
2. In a large bowl, mix the eggs and milk. Using a fork, add the fish strips to the egg mixture and stir gently to coat.
3. Put the cornmeal, bread crumbs, smoked paprika, salt, and pepper in a quart-size zip-top plastic bag. Using a fork or tongs, transfer the fish to the bag, letting the excess egg wash drip off into the bowl before transferring. Seal the bag and shake gently to completely coat each fish stick.
4. With oven mitts, carefully remove the hot baking sheet from the oven and spray it with nonstick cooking spray. Using a fork or tongs, remove the fish sticks from the bag and arrange them on the hot baking sheet, with space between them so the hot air can circulate and crisp them up.
5. Bake for 5 to 8 minutes, until gentle pressure with a fork causes the fish to flake, and serve.

Per Serving
calories: 238 | fat: 2g | protein: 22g
carbs: 28g | fiber: 1g | sodium: 494mg

Garlic Shrimp Black Bean Pasta

Prep time: 10 minutes | Cook time: 15 minutes | Serves 4

1 pound (454 g) black bean linguine or spaghetti
1 pound (454 g) fresh shrimp, peeled and deveined
4 tablespoons extra-virgin olive oil
1 onion, finely chopped
3 garlic cloves, minced
¼ cup basil, cut into strips

1. Bring a large pot of water to a boil and cook the pasta according to the package instructions.
2. In the last 5 minutes of cooking the pasta, add the shrimp to the hot water and allow them to cook for 3 to 5 minutes. Once they turn pink, take them out of the hot water, and, if you think you may have overcooked them, run them under cool water. Set aside.
3. Reserve 1 cup of the pasta cooking water and drain the noodles. In the same pan, heat the oil over medium-high heat and cook the onion and garlic for 7 to 10 minutes. Once the onion is translucent, add the pasta back in and toss well.
4. Plate the pasta, then top with shrimp and garnish with basil.

Per Serving
calories: 668 | fat: 19g | protein: 57g
carbs: 73g | fiber: 31g | sodium: 615mg

Shrimp and Veggie Pita

Prep time: 15 minutes | Cook time: 6 minutes | Serves 4

1 pound (454 g) medium shrimp, peeled and deveined
2 tablespoons olive oil
1 teaspoon dried oregano
½ teaspoon dried thyme
½ teaspoon garlic powder
¼ teaspoon onion powder
½ teaspoon salt
¼ teaspoon black pepper
4 whole wheat pitas
4 ounces (113 g) feta cheese, crumbled
1 cup shredded lettuce
1 tomato, diced
¼ cup black olives, sliced
1 lemon

1. Preheat the oven to 380ºF (193ºC).
2. In a medium bowl, combine the shrimp with the olive oil, oregano, thyme, garlic powder, onion powder, salt, and black pepper.
3. Pour shrimp in a single layer in the air fryer basket and cook for 6 to 8 minutes, or until cooked through.
4. Remove from the air fryer and divide into warmed pitas with feta, lettuce, tomato, olives, and a squeeze of lemon.

Per Serving
calories: 395 | fat: 15g | protein: 26g
carbs: 40g | fiber: 4g | sodium: 728mg

Roasted Shrimp-Gnocchi Bake

Prep time: 10 minutes | Cook time: 20 minutes | Serves 4

1 cup chopped fresh tomato
2 tablespoons extra-virgin olive oil
2 garlic cloves, minced
½ teaspoon freshly ground black pepper
¼ teaspoon crushed red pepper
1 (12-ounce / 340-g) jar roasted red peppers, drained and coarsely chopped
1 pound (454 g) fresh raw shrimp (or frozen and thawed shrimp), shells and tails removed
1 pound (454 g) frozen gnocchi (not thawed)
½ cup cubed feta cheese
⅓ cup fresh torn basil leaves

1. Preheat the oven to 425ºF (220ºC).
2. In a baking dish, mix the tomatoes, oil, garlic, black pepper, and crushed red pepper. Roast in the oven for 10 minutes.
3. Stir in the roasted peppers and shrimp. Roast for 10 more minutes, until the shrimp turn pink and white.
4. While the shrimp cooks, cook the gnocchi on the stove top according to the package directions. Drain in a colander and keep warm.
5. Remove the dish from the oven. Mix in the cooked gnocchi, feta, and basil, and serve.

Per Serving
calories: 146 | fat: 4g | protein: 23g
carbs: 1g | fiber: 0g | sodium: 1144mg

Almond-Crusted Swordfish

Prep time: 25 minutes | Cook time: 15 minutes | Serves 4

½ cup almond flour
¼ cup crushed Marcona almonds
½ to 1 teaspoon salt, divided
2 pounds (907 g) Swordfish, preferably 1 inch thick
1 large egg, beaten (optional)
¼ cup pure apple cider
¼ cup extra-virgin olive oil, plus more for frying
3 to 4 sprigs flat-leaf parsley, chopped
1 lemon, juiced
1 tablespoon Spanish paprika
5 medium baby portobello mushrooms, chopped (optional)
4 or 5 chopped scallions, both green and white parts
3 to 4 garlic cloves, peeled
¼ cup chopped pitted Kalamata olives

1. On a dinner plate, spread the flour and crushed Marcona almonds and mix in the salt. Alternately, pour the flour, almonds, and ¼ teaspoon of salt into a large plastic food storage bag. Add the fish and coat it with the flour mixture. If a thicker coat is desired, repeat this step after dipping the fish in the egg (if using).
2. In a measuring cup, combine the apple cider, ¼ cup of olive oil, parsley, lemon juice, paprika, and ¼ teaspoon of salt. Mix well and set aside.
3. In a large, heavy-bottom sauté pan or skillet, pour the olive oil to a depth of ⅛ inch and heat on medium heat. Once the oil is hot, add the fish and brown for 3 to 5 minutes, then turn the fish over and add the mushrooms (If using), scallions, garlic, and olives. Cook for an additional 3 minutes. Once the other side of the fish is brown, remove the fish from the pan and set aside.
4. Pour the cider mixture into the skillet and mix well with the vegetables. Put the fried fish into the skillet on top of the mixture and cook with sauce on medium-low heat for 10 minutes, until the fish flakes easily with a fork. Carefully remove the fish from the pan and plate. Spoon the sauce over the fish. Serve with white rice or home-fried potatoes.

Per Serving

calories: 620 | fat: 37g | protein: 63g
carbs: 10g | fiber: 5g | sodium: 644mg

Sea Scallops with White Bean Purée

Prep time: 10 minutes | Cook time: 10 minutes | Serves 2

4 tablespoons olive oil, divided
2 garlic cloves
2 teaspoons minced fresh rosemary
1 (15-ounce / 425-g) can white cannellini beans, drained and rinsed
½ cup low-sodium chicken stock
Salt, to taste
Freshly ground black pepper, to taste
6 (10 ounce / 283-g) sea scallops

1. To make the bean purée, heat 2 tablespoons of olive oil in a saucepan over medium-high heat. Add the garlic and sauté for 30 seconds, or just until it's fragrant. Don't let it burn. Add the rosemary and remove the pan from the heat.
2. Add the white beans and chicken stock to the pan, return it to the heat, and stir. Bring the beans to a boil. Reduce the heat to low and simmer for 5 minutes.
3. Transfer the beans to a blender and purée them for 30 seconds, or until they're smooth. Taste and season with salt and pepper. Let them sit in the blender with the lid on to keep them warm while you prepare the scallops.
4. Pat the scallops dry with a paper towel and season them with salt and pepper.
5. Heat the remaining 2 tablespoons of olive oil in a large sauté pan. When the oil is shimmering, add the scallops, flat-side down.
6. Cook the scallops for 2 minutes, or until they're golden on the bottom. Flip them over and cook for another 1 to 2 minutes, or until opaque and slightly firm.
7. To serve, divide the bean purée between two plates and top with the scallops.

Per Serving

calories: 465 | fat: 28g | protein: 30g
carbs: 21g | fiber: 7g | sodium: 319mg

Sea Bass Crusted with Moroccan Spices

Prep time: 15 minutes | Cook time: 40 minutes | Serves 4

1½ teaspoons ground turmeric, divided
¾ teaspoon saffron
½ teaspoon ground cumin
¼ teaspoon kosher salt
¼ teaspoon freshly ground black pepper
1½ pounds (680 g) sea bass fillets, about ½ inch thick
8 tablespoons extra-virgin olive oil, divided
8 garlic cloves, divided (4 minced cloves and 4 sliced)
6 medium baby portobello mushrooms, chopped
1 large carrot, sliced on an angle
2 sun-dried tomatoes, thinly sliced (optional)
2 tablespoons tomato paste
1 (15-ounce / 425-g) can chickpeas, drained and rinsed
1½ cups low-sodium vegetable broth
¼ cup white wine
1 tablespoon ground coriander (optional)
1 cup sliced artichoke hearts marinated in olive oil
½ cup pitted Kalamata olives
½ lemon, juiced
½ lemon, cut into thin rounds
4 to 5 rosemary sprigs or 2 tablespoons dried rosemary
Fresh cilantro, for garnish

1. In a small mixing bowl, combine 1 teaspoon turmeric and the saffron and cumin. Season with salt and pepper. Season both sides of the fish with the spice mixture. Add 3 tablespoons of olive oil and work the fish to make sure it's well coated with the spices and the olive oil.
2. In a large sauté pan or skillet, heat 2 tablespoons of olive oil over medium heat until shimmering but not smoking. Sear the top side of the sea bass for about 1 minute, or until golden. Remove and set aside.
3. In the same skillet, add the minced garlic and cook very briefly, tossing regularly, until fragrant. Add the mushrooms, carrot, sun-dried tomatoes (if using), and tomato paste. Cook for 3 to 4 minutes over medium heat, tossing frequently, until fragrant. Add the chickpeas, broth, wine, coriander (if using), and the sliced garlic. Stir in the remaining ½ teaspoon ground turmeric. Raise the heat, if needed, and bring to a boil, then lower heat to simmer. Cover part of the way and let the sauce simmer for about 20 minutes, until thickened.
4. Carefully add the seared fish to the skillet. Ladle a bit of the sauce on top of the fish. Add the artichokes, olives, lemon juice and slices, and rosemary sprigs. Cook another 10 minutes or until the fish is fully cooked and flaky. Garnish with fresh cilantro.

Per Serving
calories: 696 | fat: 41g | protein: 48g
carbs: 37g | fiber: 9g | sodium: 810mg

Sea Bass with Roasted Root Veggie

Prep time: 10 minutes | Cook time: 15 minutes | Serves 15

1 carrot, diced small
1 parsnip, diced small
1 rutabaga, diced small
¼ cup olive oil
2 teaspoons salt, divided
4 sea bass fillets
½ teaspoon onion powder
2 garlic cloves, minced
1 lemon, sliced, plus additional wedges for serving

1. Preheat the air fryer to 380ºF (193ºC).
2. In a small bowl, toss the carrot, parsnip, and rutabaga with olive oil and 1 teaspoon salt.
3. Lightly season the sea bass with the remaining 1 teaspoon of salt and the onion powder, then place it into the air fryer basket in a single layer.
4. Spread the garlic over the top of each fillet, then cover with lemon slices.
5. Pour the prepared vegetables into the basket around and on top of the fish. Roast for 15 minutes.
6. Serve with additional lemon wedges if desired.

Per Serving
calories: 299 | fat: 15g | protein: 25g
carbs: 13g | fiber: 2g | sodium: 1232mg

Olive Oil-Poached Tuna

Prep time: 5 minutes | Cook time: 45 minutes | Serves 4

1 cup extra-virgin olive oil, plus more if needed
4 (3- to 4-inch) sprigs fresh rosemary
8 (3- to 4-inch) sprigs fresh thyme
2 large garlic cloves, thinly sliced
2 (2-inch) strips lemon zest
1 teaspoon salt
½ teaspoon freshly ground black pepper
1 pound (454 g) fresh tuna steaks (about 1 inch thick)

1. Select a thick pot just large enough to fit the tuna in a single layer on the bottom. The larger the pot, the more olive oil you will need to use. Combine the olive oil, rosemary, thyme, garlic, lemon zest, salt, and pepper over medium-low heat and cook until warm and fragrant, 20 to 25 minutes, lowering the heat if it begins to smoke.
2. Remove from the heat and allow to cool for 25 to 30 minutes, until warm but not hot.
3. Add the tuna to the bottom of the pan, adding additional oil if needed so that tuna is fully submerged, and return to medium-low heat. Cook for 5 to 10 minutes, or until the oil heats back up and is warm and fragrant but not smoking. Lower the heat if it gets too hot.
4. Remove the pot from the heat and let the tuna cook in warm oil 4 to 5 minutes, to your desired level of doneness. For a tuna that is rare in the center, cook for 2 to 3 minutes.
5. Remove from the oil and serve warm, drizzling 2 to 3 tablespoons seasoned oil over the tuna.
6. To store for later use, remove the tuna from the oil and place in a container with a lid. Allow tuna and oil to cool separately. When both have cooled, remove the herb stems with a slotted spoon and pour the cooking oil over the tuna. Cover and store in the refrigerator for up to 1 week. Bring to room temperature to allow the oil to liquify before serving.

Per Serving
calories: 363 | fat: 28g | protein: 27g
carbs: 1g | fiber: 0g | sodium: 624mg

Shrimp, Mushrooms, Basil Cheese Pasta

Prep time: 10 minutes | Cook time: 10 minutes | Serves 6

1 pound (454 g) small shrimp, peeled and deveined
¼ cup plus 1 tablespoon olive oil, divided
¼ teaspoon garlic powder
¼ teaspoon cayenne
1 pound (454 g) whole grain pasta
5 garlic cloves, minced
8 ounces (227 g) baby bella mushrooms, sliced
½ cup Parmesan, plus more for serving (optional)
1 teaspoon salt
½ teaspoon black pepper
½ cup fresh basil

1. Preheat the air fryer to 380ºF (193ºC).
2. In a small bowl, combine the shrimp, 1 tablespoon olive oil, garlic powder, and cayenne. Toss to coat the shrimp.
3. Place the shrimp into the air fryer basket and roast for 5 minutes. Remove the shrimp and set aside.
4. Cook the pasta according to package directions. Once done cooking, reserve ½ cup pasta water, then drain.
5. Meanwhile, in a large skillet, heat ¼ cup of olive oil over medium heat. Add the garlic and mushrooms and cook down for 5 minutes.
6. Pour the pasta, reserved pasta water, Parmesan, salt, pepper, and basil into the skillet with the vegetable-and-oil mixture, and stir to coat the pasta.
7. Toss in the shrimp and remove from heat, then let the mixture sit for 5 minutes before serving with additional Parmesan, if desired.

Per Serving
calories: 457 | fat: 14g | protein: 25g
carbs: 60g | fiber: 6g | sodium: 411mg

Shrimp Pesto Rice Bowls

Prep time: 5 minutes | Cook time: 5 minutes | Serves 4

1 pound (454 g) medium shrimp, peeled and deveined	1 lemon, sliced
¼ cup pesto sauce	2 cups cooked wild rice pilaf

1. Preheat the air fryer to 360ºF (182ºC).
2. In a medium bowl, toss the shrimp with the pesto sauce until well coated.
3. Place the shrimp in a single layer in the air fryer basket. Put the lemon slices over the shrimp and roast for 5 minutes.
4. Remove the lemons and discard. Serve a quarter of the shrimp over ½ cup wild rice with some favorite steamed vegetables.

Per Serving

calories: 249 | fat: 10g | protein: 20g
carbs: 20g | fiber: 2g | sodium: 277mg

Salmon with Tomatoes and Olives

Prep time: 5 minutes | Cook time: 8 minutes | Serves 4

2 tablespoons olive oil	fresh dill
4 (1½-inch-thick) salmon fillets	2 Roma tomatoes, diced
½ teaspoon salt	¼ cup sliced Kalamata olives
¼ teaspoon cayenne	4 lemon slices
1 teaspoon chopped	

1. Preheat the air fryer to 380ºF (193ºC).
2. Brush the olive oil on both sides of the salmon fillets, and then season them lightly with salt, cayenne, and dill.
3. Place the fillets in a single layer in the basket of the air fryer, then layer the tomatoes and olives over the top. Top each fillet with a lemon slice.
4. Bake for 8 minutes, or until the salmon has reached an internal temperature of 145ºF (63ºC).

Per Serving

calories: 241 | fat: 15g | protein: 23g
carbs: 3g | fiber: 1g | sodium: 595mg

Golden Salmon Cakes with Tzatziki Sauce

Prep time: 15 minutes | Cook time: 11 minutes | Serves 2

For the Tzatziki Sauce:

½ cup plain Greek yogurt	cucumber
1 teaspoon dried dill	Salt, to taste
¼ cup minced	Freshly ground black pepper, to taste

For the Salmon Cakes:

6 ounces (170 g) cooked salmon	minced parsley
3 tablespoons olive oil, divided	Salt, to taste
¼ cup minced celery	Freshly ground black pepper, to taste
¼ cup minced onion	1 egg, beaten
½ teaspoon dried dill	½ cup unseasoned bread crumbs
1 tablespoon fresh	

Make the Tzatziki Sauce

1. Combine the yogurt, dill, and cucumber in a small bowl. Season with salt and pepper and set aside.

Make the Salmon Cakes

1. Remove any skin from the salmon. Place the salmon in a medium bowl and break it into small flakes with a fork. Set it aside.
2. Heat 1 tablespoon of olive oil in a nonstick skillet over medium-high heat. Add the celery and onion and sauté for 5 minutes.
3. Add the celery and onion to the salmon and stir to combine. Add the dill and parsley, and season with salt and pepper.
4. Add the beaten egg and bread crumbs and stir until mixed thoroughly.
5. Wipe the skillet clean and add the remaining 2 tablespoons of oil. Heat the pan over medium-high heat.
6. Form the salmon mixture into 4 patties, and place them two at a time into the hot pan.
7. Cook for 3 minutes per side, or until they're golden brown. Carefully flip them over with a spatula and cook for another 3 minutes on the second side.
8. Repeat with the remaining salmon cakes and serve topped with the tzatziki sauce.

Per Serving

calories: 555 | fat: 40g | protein: 31g
carbs: 18g | fiber: 1g | sodium: 303mg

Baked Trout with Lemon

Prep time: 5 minutes | Cook time: 15 minutes | Serves 4

4 trout fillets
2 tablespoons olive oil
½ teaspoon salt
1 teaspoon black pepper
2 garlic cloves, sliced
1 lemon, sliced, plus additional wedges for serving

1. Preheat the air fryer to 380ºF (193ºC).
2. Brush each fillet with olive oil on both sides and season with salt and pepper. Place the fillets in an even layer in the air fryer basket.
3. Place the sliced garlic over the tops of the trout fillets, then top the garlic with lemon slices and cook for 12 to 15 minutes, or until it has reached an internal temperature of 145ºF (63ºC).
4. Serve with fresh lemon wedges.

Per Serving
calories: 231 | fat: 12g | protein: 29g
carbs: 1g | fiber: 0g | sodium: 341mg

Sicilian Tuna and Veggie Bowl

Prep time: 10 minutes | Cook time: 16 minutes | Serves 6

1 pound (454 g) kale, chopped, center ribs removed
3 tablespoons extra-virgin olive oil
1 cup chopped onion
3 garlic cloves, minced
1 (2¼-ounce / 64-g) can sliced olives, drained
¼ cup capers
¼ teaspoon crushed red pepper
2 teaspoons sugar
2 (6-ounce / 170-g) cans tuna in olive oil, undrained
1 (15-ounce / 425-g) can cannellini beans or great northern beans, drained and rinsed
¼ teaspoon freshly ground black pepper
¼ teaspoon kosher or sea salt

1. Fill a large stockpot three-quarters full of water, and bring to a boil. Add the kale and cook for 2 minutes. (This is to make the kale less bitter.) Drain the kale in a colander and set aside.
2. Set the empty pot back on the stove over medium heat, and pour in the oil.

Add the onion and cook for 4 minutes, stirring often. Add the garlic and cook for 1 minute, stirring often. Add the olives, capers, and crushed red pepper, and cook for 1 minute, stirring often. Add the partially cooked kale and sugar, stirring until the kale is completely coated with oil. Cover the pot and cook for 8 minutes.
3. Remove the kale from the heat, mix in the tuna, beans, pepper, and salt, and serve.

Per Serving
calories: 372 | fat: 28g | protein: 8g
carbs: 22g | fiber: 7g | sodium: 452mg

Cod Fillet with Swiss Chard

Prep time: 10 minutes | Cook time: 12 minutes | Serves 4

1 teaspoon salt
½ teaspoon dried oregano
½ teaspoon dried thyme
½ teaspoon garlic powder
4 cod fillets
½ white onion, thinly sliced
2 cups Swiss chard, washed, stemmed, and torn into pieces
¼ cup olive oil
1 lemon, quartered

1. Preheat the air fryer to 380ºF (193ºC).
2. In a small bowl, whisk together the salt, oregano, thyme, and garlic powder.
3. Tear off four pieces of aluminum foil, with each sheet being large enough to envelop one cod fillet and a quarter of the vegetables.
4. Place a cod fillet in the middle of each sheet of foil, then sprinkle on all sides with the spice mixture.
5. In each foil packet, place a quarter of the onion slices and ½ cup Swiss chard, then drizzle 1 tablespoon olive oil and squeeze ¼ lemon over the contents of each foil packet.
6. Fold and seal the sides of the foil packets and then place them into the air fryer basket. Steam for 12 minutes.
7. Remove from the basket, and carefully open each packet to avoid a steam burn.

Per Serving
calories: 252 | fat: 13g | protein: 26g
carbs: 4g | fiber: 1g | sodium: 641mg

Salmon with Broccoli Rabe and Cannellini Beans

Prep time: 10 minutes | Cook time: 11 minutes | Serves 4

2 tablespoons extra-virgin olive oil, plus extra for drizzling
4 garlic cloves, sliced thin
½ cup chicken or vegetable broth
¼ teaspoon red pepper flakes
1 lemon, sliced ¼ inch thick, plus lemon wedges for serving
4 (6-ounce / 170-g) skinless salmon fillets, 1½ inches thick
½ teaspoon table salt
¼ teaspoon pepper
1 pound (454 g) broccoli rabe, trimmed and cut into 1-inch pieces
1 (15-ounce / 425-g) can cannellini beans, rinsed

1. Using highest sauté function, cook oil and garlic in Instant Pot until garlic is fragrant and light golden brown, about 3 minutes. Using slotted spoon, transfer garlic to paper towel–lined plate and season with salt to taste; set aside for serving. Turn off Instant Pot, then stir in broth and pepper flakes.
2. Fold sheet of aluminum foil into 16 by 6-inch sling. Arrange lemon slices widthwise in 2 rows across center of sling. Sprinkle flesh side of salmon with salt and pepper, then arrange skinned side down on top of lemon slices. Using sling, lower salmon into Instant Pot; allow narrow edges of sling to rest along sides of insert. Lock lid in place and close pressure release valve. Select high pressure cook function and cook for 3 minutes.
3. Turn off Instant Pot and quick-release pressure. Carefully remove lid, allowing steam to escape away from you. Using sling, transfer salmon to large plate. Tent with foil and let rest while preparing broccoli rabe mixture.
4. Stir broccoli rabe and beans into cooking liquid, partially cover, and cook, using highest sauté function, until broccoli rabe is tender, about 5 minutes. Season with salt and pepper to taste. Gently lift and tilt salmon fillets with spatula to remove lemon slices. Serve salmon with broccoli rabe mixture and lemon wedges, sprinkling individual portions with garlic chips and drizzling with extra oil.

Per Serving
calories: 510 | fat: 5g | protein: 43g
carbs: 15g | fiber: 5g | sodium: 232mg

Tilapia Fillet with Onion and Avocado

Prep time: 5 minutes | Cook time: 3 minutes | Serves 4

1 tablespoon extra-virgin olive oil
1 tablespoon freshly squeezed orange juice
¼ teaspoon kosher or sea salt
4 (4-ounce/ 113-g) tilapia fillets, more oblong than square, skin-on or skinned
¼ cup chopped red onion
1 avocado, pitted, skinned, and sliced

1. In a 9-inch glass pie dish, use a fork to mix together the oil, orange juice, and salt. Working with one fillet at a time, place each in the pie dish and turn to coat on all sides. Arrange the fillets in a wagon-wheel formation, so that one end of each fillet is in the center of the dish and the other end is temporarily draped over the edge of the dish. Top each fillet with 1 tablespoon of onion, then fold the end of the fillet that's hanging over the edge in half over the onion. When finished, you should have 4 folded-over fillets with the fold against the outer edge of the dish and the ends all in the center.
2. Cover the dish with plastic wrap, leaving a small part open at the edge to vent the steam. Microwave on high for about 3 minutes. The fish is done when it just begins to separate into flakes (chunks) when pressed gently with a fork.
3. Top the fillets with the avocado and serve.

Per Serving
calories: 210 | fat: 10g | protein: 25g
carbs: 5g | fiber: 3g | sodium: 240mg

Cod with Green Salad and Dukkah

Prep time: 10 minutes | Cook time: 8 minutes | Serves 4

¼ cup extra-virgin olive oil, divided, plus extra for drizzling
1 shallot, sliced thin
2 garlic cloves, minced
1½ pounds (680 g) small beets, scrubbed, trimmed, and cut into ½-inch wedges
½ cup chicken or vegetable broth
1 tablespoon dukkah, plus extra for sprinkling
¼ teaspoon table salt
4 (6-ounce / 170-g) skinless cod fillets, 1½ inches thick
1 tablespoon lemon juice
2 ounces (57 g) baby arugula

1. Using highest sauté function, heat 1 tablespoon oil in Instant Pot until shimmering. Add shallot and cook until softened, about 2 minutes. Stir in garlic and cook until fragrant, about 30 seconds. Stir in beets and broth. Lock lid in place and close pressure release valve. Select high pressure cook function and cook for 3 minutes. Turn off Instant Pot and quick-release pressure. Carefully remove lid, allowing steam to escape away from you.
2. Fold sheet of aluminum foil into 16 by 6-inch sling. Combine 2 tablespoons oil, dukkah, and salt in bowl, then brush cod with oil mixture. Arrange cod skinned side down in center of sling. Using sling, lower cod into Instant Pot; allow narrow edges of sling to rest along sides of insert. Lock lid in place and close pressure release valve. Select high pressure cook function and cook for 2 minutes.
3. Turn off Instant Pot and quick-release pressure. Carefully remove lid, allowing steam to escape away from you. Using sling, transfer cod to large plate. Tent with foil and let rest while finishing beet salad.
4. Combine lemon juice and remaining 1 tablespoon oil in large bowl. Using slotted spoon, transfer beets to bowl with oil mixture. Add arugula and gently toss to combine. Season with salt and pepper to taste. Serve cod with salad, sprinkling individual portions with extra dukkah and drizzling with extra oil.

Per Serving
calories: 340 | fat: 15g | protein: 33g
carbs: 14g | fiber: 3g | sodium: 231mg

Pressure-Cooked Mussels

Prep time: 10 minutes | Cook time: 6 minutes | Serves 4

1 tablespoon extra-virgin olive oil, plus extra for drizzling
1 fennel bulb, 1 tablespoon fronds minced, stalks discarded, bulb halved, cored, and sliced thin
1 leek, ends trimmed, leek halved lengthwise, sliced
1 inch thick, and washed thoroughly
4 garlic cloves, minced
3 sprigs fresh thyme
¼ teaspoon red pepper flakes
½ cup dry white wine
3 pounds (1.4 kg) mussels, scrubbed and debearded

1. Using highest sauté function, heat oil in Instant Pot until shimmering. Add fennel and leek and cook until softened, about 5 minutes. Stir in garlic, thyme sprigs, and pepper flakes and cook until fragrant, about 30 seconds. Stir in wine, then add mussels.
2. Lock lid in place and close pressure release valve. Select high pressure cook function and set cook time for 0 minutes. Once Instant Pot has reached pressure, immediately turn off pot and quick-release pressure. Carefully remove lid, allowing steam to escape away from you.
3. Discard thyme sprigs and any mussels that have not opened. Transfer mussels to individual serving bowls, sprinkle with fennel fronds, and drizzle with extra oil. Serve.

Per Serving
calories: 380 | fat: 10g | protein: 42g
carbs: 22g | fiber: 1g | sodium: 342mg

Fish Fillet on Lemons

Prep time: 5 minutes | Cook time: 6 minutes | Serves 4

4 (4-ounce/ 113-g) fish fillets, such as tilapia, salmon, catfish, cod, or your favorite fish
Nonstick cooking spray
3 to 4 medium lemons
1 tablespoon extra-virgin olive oil
¼ teaspoon freshly ground black pepper
¼ teaspoon kosher or sea salt

1. Using paper towels, pat the fillets dry and let stand at room temperature for 10 minutes. Meanwhile, coat the cold cooking grate of the grill with nonstick cooking spray, and preheat the grill to 400ºF (205ºC), or medium-high heat. Or preheat a grill pan over medium-high heat on the stove top.
2. Cut one lemon in half and set half aside. Slice the remaining half of that lemon and the remaining lemons into ¼-inch-thick slices. (You should have about 12 to 16 lemon slices.) Into a small bowl, squeeze 1 tablespoon of juice out of the reserved lemon half.
3. Add the oil to the bowl with the lemon juice, and mix well. Brush both sides of the fish with the oil mixture, and sprinkle evenly with pepper and salt.
4. Carefully place the lemon slices on the grill (or the grill pan), arranging 3 to 4 slices together in the shape of a fish fillet, and repeat with the remaining slices. Place the fish fillets directly on top of the lemon slices, and grill with the lid closed. (If you're grilling on the stove top, cover with a large pot lid or aluminum foil.) Turn the fish halfway through the cooking time only if the fillets are more than half an inch thick. The fish is done and ready to serve when it just begins to separate into flakes (chunks) when pressed gently with a fork.

Per Serving

calories: 208 | fat: 11g | protein: 21g
carbs: 2g | fiber: 0g | sodium: 249mg

Oregano Shrimp Puttanesca

Prep time: 10 minutes | Cook time: 9 minutes | Serves 4

2 tablespoons extra-virgin olive oil
3 anchovy fillets, drained and chopped, or 1½ teaspoons anchovy paste
3 garlic cloves, minced
½ teaspoon crushed red pepper
1 (14½-ounce / 411-g) can low-sodium or no-salt-added diced tomatoes, undrained
1 (2¼-ounce / 64-g) can sliced black olives, drained
2 tablespoons capers
1 tablespoon chopped fresh oregano or 1 teaspoon dried oregano
1 pound fresh raw shrimp (or frozen and thawed shrimp), shells and tails removed

1. In a large skillet over medium heat, heat the oil. Mix in the anchovies, garlic, and crushed red pepper. Cook for 3 minutes, stirring frequently and mashing up the anchovies with a wooden spoon, until they have melted into the oil.
2. Stir in the tomatoes with their juices, olives, capers, and oregano. Turn up the heat to medium-high, and bring to a simmer.
3. When the sauce is lightly bubbling, stir in the shrimp. Reduce the heat to medium, and cook the shrimp for 6 to 8 minutes, or until they turn pink and white, stirring occasionally, and serve.

Per Serving

calories: 362 | fat: 12g | protein: 30g
carbs: 31g | fiber: 1g | sodium: 1463mg

Hake Fillet in Saffron Broth

Prep time: 15 minutes | Cook time: 9 minutes | Serves 4

2 tablespoons extra-virgin olive oil, divided, plus extra for drizzling
1 onion, chopped
4 ounces (113 g) Spanish-style chorizo sausage, sliced ¼ inch thick
4 garlic cloves, minced
1 (8-ounce / 227-g) bottle clam juice
¾ cup water
½ cup dry white wine
8 ounces (227 g) small red potatoes, unpeeled, quartered
¼ teaspoon saffron threads, crumbled
1 bay leaf
4 (6-ounce / 170-g) skinless hake fillets, 1½ inches thick
½ teaspoon table salt
¼ teaspoon pepper
2 tablespoons minced fresh parsley

1. Using highest sauté function, heat 1 tablespoon oil in Instant Pot until shimmering. Add onion and chorizo and cook until onion is softened and lightly browned, 5 to 7 minutes. Stir in garlic and cook until fragrant, about 30 seconds. Stir in clam juice, water, and wine, scraping up any browned bits. Turn off Instant Pot, then stir in potatoes, saffron, and bay leaf.
2. Fold sheet of aluminum foil into 16 by 6-inch sling. Brush hake with remaining 1 tablespoon oil and sprinkle with salt and pepper. Arrange hake skinned side down in center of sling. Using sling, lower hake into Instant Pot on top of potato mixture; allow narrow edges of sling to rest along sides of insert. Lock lid in place and close pressure release valve. Select high pressure cook function and cook for 3 minutes.
3. Turn off Instant Pot and quick-release pressure. Carefully remove lid, allowing steam to escape away from you. Using sling, transfer hake to large plate. Tent with aluminum foil and let rest while finishing potato mixture.
4. Discard bay leaf. Stir parsley into potato mixture and season with salt to taste. Serve cod with potato mixture and broth, drizzling individual portions with extra oil.

Per Serving
calories: 410 | fat: 18g | protein: 39g | carbs: 14g | fiber: 1g | sodium: 287mg

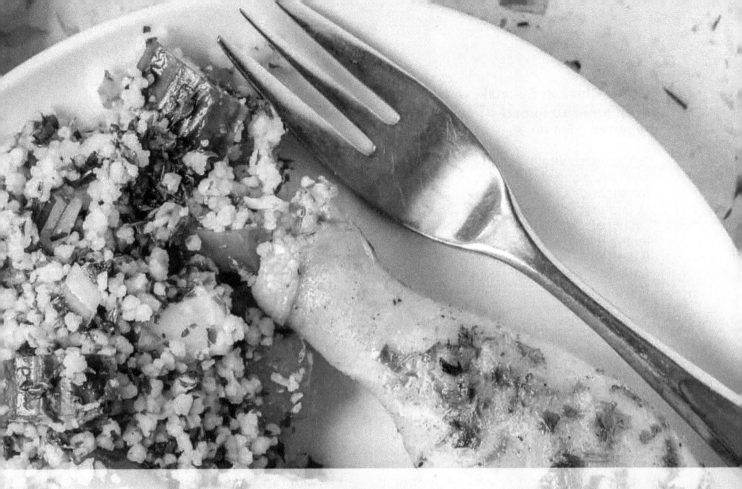
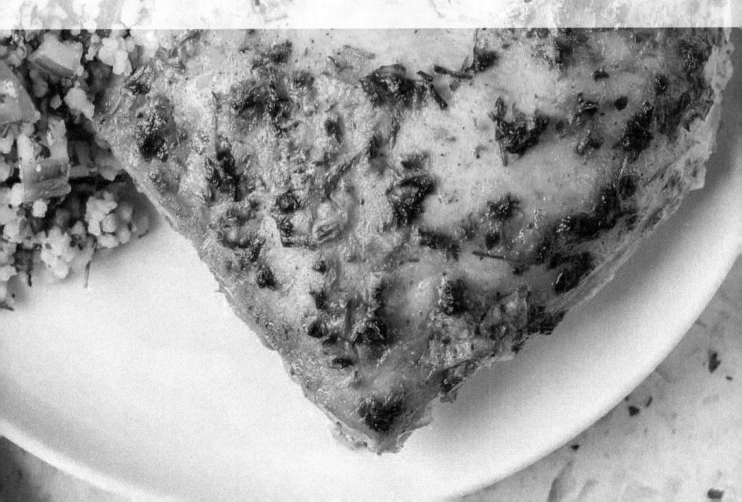

Chapter 8 Poultry

Greek Chicken Souvlaki with Tzatziki

Prep time: 10 minutes | Cook time: 8 minutes | Serves 4

½ cup extra-virgin olive oil, plus extra for serving
¼ cup dry white wine (optional; add extra lemon juice instead, if desired)
6 garlic cloves, finely minced
Zest and juice of 1 lemon
1 tablespoon dried oregano
1 teaspoon dried rosemary
½ teaspoons salt
½ teaspoon freshly ground black pepper
1 pound (454 g) boneless, skinless chicken thighs, cut into 1½-inch chunks
1 cup tzatziki, for serving

1. In a large glass bowl or resealable plastic bag, combine the olive oil, white wine (if using), garlic, lemon zest and juice, oregano, rosemary, salt, and pepper and whisk or shake to combine well. Add the chicken to the marinade and toss to coat. Cover or seal and marinate in the refrigerator for at least 1 hour, or up to 24 hours.
2. In a bowl, submerge wooden skewers in water and soak for at least 30 minutes before using.
3. To cook, heat the grill to medium-high heat. Thread the marinated chicken on the soaked skewers, reserving the marinade.
4. Grill until cooked through, flipping occasionally so that the chicken cooks evenly, 5 to 8 minutes. Remove and keep warm.
5. Bring the reserved marinade to a boil in a small saucepan. Reduce the heat to low and simmer 3 to 5 minutes.
6. Serve chicken skewers drizzled with hot marinade, adding more olive oil if desired, and tzatziki.

Per Serving
calories: 493 | fat: 45g | protein: 19g
carbs: 3g | fiber: 0g | sodium: 385mg

Feta Stuffed Chicken Breasts

Prep time: 10 minutes | Cook time: 20 minutes | Serves 4

$\frac{1}{3}$ cup cooked brown rice
1 teaspoon shawarma seasoning
4 (6-ounce / 170-g) boneless skinless chicken breasts
1 tablespoon harissa
3 tablespoons extra-virgin olive oil,
divided
Salt and freshly ground black pepper, to taste
4 small dried apricots, halved
$\frac{1}{3}$ cup crumbled feta
1 tablespoon chopped fresh parsley

1. Preheat the oven to 375ºF (190ºC).
2. In a medium bowl, mix the rice and shawarma seasoning and set aside.
3. Butterfly the chicken breasts by slicing them almost in half, starting at the thickest part and folding them open like a book.
4. In a small bowl, mix the harissa with 1 tablespoon of olive oil. Brush the chicken with the harissa oil and season with salt and pepper. The harissa adds a nice heat, so feel free to add a thicker coating for more spice.
5. Onto one side of each chicken breast, spoon 1 to 2 tablespoons of rice, then layer 2 apricot halves in each breast. Divide the feta between the chicken breasts and fold the other side over the filling to close.
6. In an oven-safe sauté pan or skillet, heat the remaining 2 tablespoons of olive oil and sear the breast for 2 minutes on each side, then place the pan into the oven for 15 minutes, or until fully cooked and juices run clear. Serve, garnished with parsley.

Per Serving
calories: 321 | fat: 17g | protein: 37g
carbs: 8g | fiber: 1g | sodium: 410mg

Poached Chicken Breast with Romesco Sauce

Prep time: 10 minutes | Cook time: 12 minutes | Serves 6

1½ pounds (680 g) boneless, skinless chicken breasts, cut into 6 pieces
1 carrot, halved
1 celery stalk, halved
½ onion, halved
2 garlic cloves, smashed
3 sprigs fresh thyme or rosemary
1 cup romesco sauce
2 tablespoons chopped fresh flat-leaf (Italian) parsley
¼ teaspoon freshly ground black pepper

1. Put the chicken in a medium saucepan. Fill with water until there's about one inch of liquid above the chicken. Add the carrot, celery, onion, garlic, and thyme. Cover and bring it to a boil. Reduce the heat to low (keeping it covered), and cook for 12 to 15 minutes, or until the internal temperature of the chicken measures 165ºF (74ºC) on a meat thermometer and any juices run clear.
2. Remove the chicken from the water and let sit for 5 minutes.
3. When you're ready to serve, spread ¾ cup of romesco sauce on the bottom of a serving platter. Arrange the chicken breasts on top, and drizzle with the remaining romesco sauce. Sprinkle the tops with parsley and pepper.

Per Serving
calories: 270 | fat: 10g | protein: 13g
carbs: 31g | fiber: 2g | sodium: 647mg

Chicken Sausage and Tomato with Farro

Prep time: 10 minutes | Cook time: 45 minutes | Serves 2

1 tablespoon olive oil
½ medium onion, diced
¼ cup julienned sun-dried tomatoes packed in olive oil and herbs
8 ounces (227 g) hot Italian chicken sausage, removed
from the casing
¾ cup farro
1½ cups low-sodium chicken stock
2 cups loosely packed arugula
4 to 5 large fresh basil leaves, sliced thin
Salt, to taste

1. Heat the olive oil in a sauté pan over medium-high heat. Add the onion and sauté for 5 minutes. Add the sun-dried tomatoes and chicken sausage, stirring to break up the sausage. Cook for 7 minutes, or until the sausage is no longer pink.
2. Stir in the farro. Let it toast for 3 minutes, stirring occasionally.
3. Add the chicken stock and bring the mixture to a boil. Cover the pan and reduce the heat to medium-low. Let it simmer for 30 minutes, or until the farro is tender.
4. Stir in the arugula and let it wilt slightly. Add the basil, and season with salt.

Per Serving
calories: 491 | fat: 18g | protein: 31g
carbs: 53g | fiber: 6g | sodium: 765mg

Yogurt-Marinated Chicken

Prep time: 15 minutes | Cook time: 30 minutes | Serves 2

½ cup plain Greek yogurt
3 garlic cloves, minced
2 tablespoons minced fresh oregano (or 1 tablespoon dried
oregano)
Zest of 1 lemon
1 tablespoon olive oil
½ teaspoon salt
2 (4-ounce / 113-g) boneless, skinless chicken breasts

1. In a medium bowl, add the yogurt, garlic, oregano, lemon zest, olive oil, and salt and stir to combine. If the yogurt is very thick, you may need to add a few tablespoons of water or a squeeze of lemon juice to thin it a bit.
2. Add the chicken to the bowl and toss it in the marinade to coat it well. Cover and refrigerate the chicken for at least 30 minutes or up to overnight.
3. Preheat the oven to 350ºF (180ºC) and set the rack to the middle position.
4. Place the chicken in a baking dish and roast for 30 minutes, or until chicken reaches an internal temperature of 165ºF (74ºC).

Per Serving
calories: 255 | fat: 13g | protein: 29g
carbs: 8g | fiber: 2g | sodium: 694mg

Spatchcock Chicken with Lemon and Rosemary

Prep time: 20 minutes | Cook time: 45 minutes | Serves 6 to 8

½ cup extra-virgin olive oil, divided
1 (3- to 4-pound / 1.4- to 1.8-kg) roasting chicken
8 garlic cloves, roughly chopped
2 to 4 tablespoons chopped fresh

rosemary
2 teaspoons salt, divided
1 teaspoon freshly ground black pepper, divided
2 lemons, thinly sliced

1. Preheat the oven to 425ºF (220ºC).
2. Pour 2 tablespoons olive oil in the bottom of a 9-by-13-inch baking dish or rimmed baking sheet and swirl to coat the bottom.
3. To spatchcock the bird, place the whole chicken breast-side down on a large work surface. Using a very sharp knife, cut along the backbone, starting at the tail end and working your way up to the neck. Pull apart the two sides, opening up the chicken. Flip it over, breast-side up, pressing down with your hands to flatten the bird. Transfer to the prepared baking dish.
4. Loosen the skin over the breasts and thighs by cutting a small incision and sticking one or two fingers inside to pull the skin away from the meat without removing it.
5. To prepare the filling, in a small bowl, combine ¼ cup olive oil, garlic, rosemary, 1 teaspoon salt, and ½ teaspoon pepper and whisk together.
6. Rub the garlic-herb oil evenly under the skin of each breast and each thigh. Add the lemon slices evenly to the same areas.
7. Whisk together the remaining 2 tablespoons olive oil, 1 teaspoon salt, and ½ teaspoon pepper and rub over the outside of the chicken.
8. Place in the oven, uncovered, and roast for 45 minutes, or until cooked through and golden brown. Allow to rest 5 minutes before carving to serve.

Per Serving

calories: 435 | fat: 34g | protein: 28g
carbs: 2g | fiber: 0g | sodium: 879mg

Lemon Chicken Thighs with Vegetables

Prep time: 15 minutes | Cook time: 45 minutes | Serves 4

6 tablespoons extra-virgin olive oil, divided
4 large garlic cloves, crushed
1 tablespoon dried basil
1 tablespoon dried parsley
1 tablespoon salt
½ tablespoon thyme
4 skin-on, bone-in chicken thighs

6 medium portobello mushrooms, quartered
1 large zucchini, sliced
1 large carrot, thinly sliced
⅛ cup pitted Kalamata olives
8 pieces sun-dried tomatoes (optional)
½ cup dry white wine
1 lemon, sliced

1. In a small bowl, combine 4 tablespoons of olive oil, the garlic cloves, basil, parsley, salt, and thyme. Store half of the marinade in a jar and, in a bowl, combine the remaining half to marinate the chicken thighs for about 30 minutes.
2. Preheat the oven to 425ºF (220ºC).
3. In a large skillet or oven-safe pan, heat the remaining 2 tablespoons of olive oil over medium-high heat. Sear the chicken for 3 to 5 minutes on each side until golden brown, and set aside.
4. In the same pan, sauté portobello mushrooms, zucchini, and carrot for about 5 minutes, or until lightly browned.
5. Add the chicken thighs, olives, and sun-dried tomatoes (if using). Pour the wine over the chicken thighs.
6. Cover the pan and cook for about 10 minutes over medium-low heat.
7. Uncover the pan and transfer it to the oven. Cook for 15 more minutes, or until the chicken skin is crispy and the juices run clear. Top with lemon slices.

Per Serving

calories: 544 | fat: 41g | protein: 28g
carbs: 20g | fiber: 11g | sodium: 1848mg

Chicken Skewers with Veggies
Prep time: 30 minutes | Cook time: 25 minutes | Serves 4

¼ cup olive oil
1 teaspoon garlic powder
1 teaspoon onion powder
1 teaspoon ground cumin
½ teaspoon dried oregano
½ teaspoon dried basil
¼ cup lemon juice
1 tablespoon apple cider vinegar
Olive oil cooking spray
1 pound (454 g) boneless skinless chicken thighs, cut into 1-inch pieces
1 red bell pepper, cut into 1-inch pieces
1 red onion, cut into 1-inch pieces
1 zucchini, cut into 1-inch pieces
12 cherry tomatoes

1. In a large bowl, mix together the olive oil, garlic powder, onion powder, cumin, oregano, basil, lemon juice, and apple cider vinegar.
2. Spray six skewers with olive oil cooking spray.
3. On each skewer, slide on a piece of chicken, then a piece of bell pepper, onion, zucchini, and finally a tomato and then repeat. Each skewer should have at least two pieces of each item.
4. Once all of the skewers are prepared, place them in a 9-by-13-inch baking dish and pour the olive oil marinade over the top of the skewers. Turn each skewer so that all sides of the chicken and vegetables are coated.
5. Cover the dish with plastic wrap and place it in the refrigerator for 30 minutes.
6. After 30 minutes, preheat the air fryer to 380ºF (193ºC). (If using a grill attachment, make sure it is inside the air fryer during preheating.)
7. Remove the skewers from the marinade and lay them in a single layer in the air fryer basket. If the air fryer has a grill attachment, you can also lay them on this instead.
8. Cook for 10 minutes. Rotate the kebabs, then cook them for 15 minutes more.
9. Remove the skewers from the air fryer and let them rest for 5 minutes before serving.

Per Serving
calories: 304 | fat: 17g | protein: 27g
carbs: 10g | fiber: 3g | sodium: 62mg

Greek Lemon Chicken Kebabs
Prep time: 15 minutes | Cook time: 20 minutes | Serves 2

½ cup extra-virgin olive oil, divided
½ large lemon, juiced
2 garlic cloves, minced
½ teaspoon za'atar seasoning
Salt and freshly ground black pepper, to taste
1 pound (454 g) boneless skinless chicken breasts, cut
into 1¼-inch cubes
1 large red bell pepper, cut into 1¼-inch pieces
2 small zucchini (nearly 1 pound / 454 g), cut into rounds slightly under ½ inch thick
2 large shallots, diced into quarters
Tzatziki sauce, for serving

1. In a bowl, whisk together ⅓ cup of olive oil, lemon juice, garlic, za'atar, salt, and pepper.
2. Put the chicken in a medium bowl and pour the olive oil mixture over the chicken. Press the chicken into the marinade. Cover and refrigerate for 45 minutes. While the chicken marinates, soak the wooden skewers in water for 30 minutes.
3. Drizzle and toss the pepper, zucchini, and shallots with the remaining 2½ tablespoons of olive oil and season lightly with salt.
4. Preheat the oven to 500ºF (260ºC) and put a baking sheet in the oven to heat.
5. On each skewer, thread a red bell pepper, zucchini, shallot and 2 chicken pieces and repeat twice. Put the kebabs onto the hot baking sheet and cook for 7 to 9 minutes, or until the chicken is cooked through. Rotate once halfway through cooking. Serve the kebabs warm with the tzatziki sauce.

Per Serving (2 kebabs)
calories: 825 | fat: 59g | protein: 51g
carbs: 31g | fiber: 5g | sodium: 379mg

Chicken, Mushrooms, and Tarragon Pasta

Prep time: 15 minutes | Cook time: 15 minutes | Serves 2

2 tablespoons olive oil, divided
½ medium onion, minced
4 ounces (113 g) baby bella (cremini) mushrooms, sliced
2 small garlic cloves, minced
8 ounces (227 g) chicken cutlets
2 teaspoons tomato

paste
2 teaspoons dried tarragon
2 cups low-sodium chicken stock
6 ounces (170 g) pappardelle pasta
¼ cup plain full-fat Greek yogurt
Salt, to taste
Freshly ground black pepper, to taste

1. Heat 1 tablespoon of the olive oil in a sauté pan over medium-high heat. Add the onion and mushrooms and sauté for 5 minutes. Add the garlic and cook for 1 minute more.
2. Move the vegetables to the edges of the pan and add the remaining 1 tablespoon of olive oil to the center of the pan. Place the cutlets in the center and let them cook for about 3 minutes, or until they lift up easily and are golden brown on the bottom.
3. Flip the chicken and cook for another 3 minutes.
4. Mix in the tomato paste and tarragon. Add the chicken stock and stir well to combine everything. Bring the stock to a boil.
5. Add the pappardelle. Break up the pasta if needed to fit into the pan. Stir the noodles so they don't stick to the bottom of the pan.
6. Cover the sauté pan and reduce the heat to medium-low. Let the chicken and noodles simmer for 15 minutes, stirring occasionally, until the pasta is cooked and the liquid is mostly absorbed. If the liquid absorbs too quickly and the pasta isn't cooked, add more water or chicken stock, about ¼ cup at a time as needed.
7. Remove the pan from the heat.
8. Stir 2 tablespoons of the hot liquid from the pan into the yogurt. Pour the tempered yogurt into the pan and stir well to mix it into the sauce. Season with salt and pepper.
9. The sauce will tighten up as it cools, so if it seems too thick, add a few tablespoons of water.

Per Serving
calories: 556 | fat: 17g | protein: 42g
carbs: 56g | fiber: 1g | sodium: 190mg

Tahini Chicken Rice Bowls with Apricots

Prep time: 15 minutes | Cook time: 15 minutes | Serves 4

1 cup uncooked instant brown rice
¼ cup tahini or peanut butter (tahini for nut-free)
¼ cup 2% plain Greek yogurt
2 tablespoons chopped scallions, green and white parts
1 tablespoon freshly squeezed lemon juice
1 tablespoon water
1 teaspoon ground cumin

¾ teaspoon ground cinnamon
¼ teaspoon kosher or sea salt
2 cups chopped cooked chicken breast
½ cup chopped dried apricots
2 cups peeled and chopped seedless cucumber
4 teaspoons sesame seeds
Fresh mint leaves, for serving (optional)

1. Cook the brown rice according to the package instructions.
2. While the rice is cooking, in a medium bowl, mix together the tahini, yogurt, scallions, lemon juice, water, cumin, cinnamon, and salt. Transfer half the tahini mixture to another medium bowl. Mix the chicken into the first bowl.
3. When the rice is done, mix it into the second bowl of tahini (the one without the chicken).
4. To assemble, divide the chicken among four bowls. Spoon the rice mixture next to the chicken in each bowl. Next to the chicken, place the dried apricots, and in the remaining empty section, add the cucumbers. Sprinkle with sesame seeds, and top with mint, if desired, and serve.

Per Serving
calories: 335 | fat: 10g | protein: 31g
carbs: 30g | fiber: 3g | sodium: 345mg

Chicken Thigh with Roasted Artichokes

Prep time: 5 minutes | Cook time: 20 minutes | Serves 4

2 large lemons
3 tablespoons extra-virgin olive oil, divided
½ teaspoon kosher or sea salt
2 large artichokes
4 (6-ounce / 170-g) bone-in, skin-on chicken thighs

1. Put a large, rimmed baking sheet in the oven. Preheat the oven to 450°F (235°C) with the pan inside. Tear off four sheets of aluminum foil about 8-by-10 inches each; set aside.
2. Using a Microplane or citrus zester, zest 1 lemon into a large bowl. Halve both lemons and squeeze all the juice into the bowl with the zest. Whisk in 2 tablespoons of oil and the salt. Set aside.
3. Rinse the artichokes with cool water, and dry with a clean towel. Using a sharp knife, cut about 1½ inches off the tip of each artichoke. Cut about ¼ inch off each stem. Halve each artichoke lengthwise so each piece has equal amounts of stem. Immediately plunge the artichoke halves into the lemon juice and oil mixture (to prevent browning) and turn to coat on all sides. Lay one artichoke half flat-side down in the center of a sheet of aluminum foil, and close up loosely to make a foil packet. Repeat the process with the remaining three artichoke halves. Set the packets aside.
4. Put the chicken in the remaining lemon juice mixture and turn to coat.
5. Using oven mitts, carefully remove the hot baking sheet from the oven and pour on the remaining tablespoon of oil; tilt the pan to coat. Carefully arrange the chicken, skin-side down, on the hot baking sheet. Place the artichoke packets, flat-side down, on the baking sheet as well. (Arrange the artichoke packets and chicken with space between them so air can circulate around them.)
6. Roast for 20 minutes, or until the internal temperature of the chicken measures 165°F (74°C) on a meat thermometer and any juices run clear. Before serving, check the artichokes for doneness by pulling on a leaf. If it comes out easily, the artichoke is ready.

Per Serving

calories: 832 | fat: 79g | protein: 19g
carbs: 11g | fiber: 4g | sodium: 544mg

Moroccan Chicken Thighs and Vegetable Tagine

Prep time: 15 minutes | Cook time: 52 minutes | Serves 6

½ cup extra-virgin olive oil, divided
1½ pounds (680 g) boneless skinless chicken thighs, cut into 1-inch chunks
1½ teaspoons salt, divided
½ teaspoon freshly ground black pepper
1 small red onion, chopped
1 red bell pepper, cut into 1-inch squares
2 medium tomatoes, chopped or 1½
cups diced canned tomatoes
1 cup water
2 medium zucchini, sliced into ¼-inch-thick half moons
1 cup pitted halved olives (Kalamata or Spanish green work nicely)
¼ cup chopped fresh cilantro or flat-leaf Italian parsley
Riced cauliflower or sautéed spinach, for serving

1. In a Dutch oven or large rimmed skillet, heat ¼ cup olive oil over medium-high heat.
2. Season the chicken with 1 teaspoon salt and pepper and sauté until just browned on all sides, 6 to 8 minutes.
3. Add the onions and peppers and sauté until wilted, another 6 to 8 minutes.
4. Add the chopped tomatoes and water, bring to a boil, and reduce the heat to low. Cover and simmer over low heat until the meat is cooked through and very tender, 30 to 45 minutes.
5. Add the remaining ¼ cup olive oil, zucchini, olives, and cilantro, stirring to combine. Continue to cook over low heat, uncovered, until the zucchini is tender, about 10 minutes.
6. Serve warm over riced cauliflower or atop a bed of sautéed spinach.

Per Serving

calories: 358 | fat: 24g | protein: 25g
carbs: 8g | fiber: 3g | sodium: 977mg

Chicken Piccata with Mushrooms and Parsley

Prep time: 15 minutes | Cook time: 17 minutes | Serves 4

1 pound (454 g) thinly sliced chicken breasts
1½ teaspoons salt, divided
½ teaspoon freshly ground black pepper
¼ cup ground flaxseed
2 tablespoons almond flour
8 tablespoons extra-virgin olive oil, divided
4 tablespoons butter, divided (optional)
2 cups sliced mushrooms
½ cup dry white wine or chicken stock
¼ cup freshly squeezed lemon juice
¼ cup roughly chopped capers
Zucchini noodles, for serving
¼ cup chopped fresh flat-leaf Italian parsley, for garnish

1. Season the chicken with 1 teaspoon salt and the pepper. On a plate, combine the ground flaxseed and almond flour and dredge each chicken breast in the mixture. Set aside.
2. In a large skillet, heat 4 tablespoons olive oil and 1 tablespoon butter over medium-high heat. Working in batches if necessary, brown the chicken, 3 to 4 minutes per side. Remove from the skillet and keep warm.
3. Add the remaining 4 tablespoons olive oil and 1 tablespoon butter to the skillet along with mushrooms and sauté over medium heat until just tender, 6 to 8 minutes.
4. Add the white wine, lemon juice, capers, and remaining ½ teaspoon salt to the skillet and bring to a boil, whisking to incorporate any little browned bits that have stuck to the bottom of the skillet. Reduce the heat to low and whisk in the final 2 tablespoons butter.
5. Return the browned chicken to skillet, cover, and simmer over low heat until the chicken is cooked through and the sauce has thickened, 5 to 6 more minutes.
6. Serve chicken and mushrooms warm over zucchini noodles, spooning the mushroom sauce over top and garnishing with chopped parsley.

Per Serving
calories: 538 | fat: 43g | protein: 30g
carbs: 8g | fiber: 3g | sodium: 1127mg

Grilled Chicken and Zucchini Kebabs

Prep time: 10 minutes | Cook time: 20 minutes | Serves 4

¼ cup extra-virgin olive oil
2 tablespoons balsamic vinegar
1 teaspoon dried oregano, crushed between your fingers
1 pound (454 g) boneless, skinless chicken breasts, cut into 1½-inch pieces
2 medium zucchini, cut into 1-inch pieces
½ cup Kalamata olives, pitted and halved
2 tablespoons olive brine
¼ cup torn fresh basil leaves
Nonstick cooking spray
Special Equipment: 14 to 15 (12-inch) wooden skewers, soaked for at least 30 minutes

1. Spray the grill grates with nonstick cooking spray. Preheat the grill to medium-high heat.
2. In a small bowl, whisk together the olive oil, vinegar, and oregano. Divide the marinade between two large plastic zip-top bags.
3. Add the chicken to one bag and the zucchini to another. Seal and massage the marinade into both the chicken and zucchini.
4. Thread the chicken onto 6 wooden skewers. Thread the zucchini onto 8 or 9 wooden skewers.
5. Cook the kebabs in batches on the grill for 5 minutes, flip, and grill for 5 minutes more, or until any chicken juices run clear.
6. Remove the chicken and zucchini from the skewers to a large serving bowl. Toss with the olives, olive brine, and basil and serve.

Per Serving
calories: 283 | fat: 15g | protein: 11g
carbs: 26g | fiber: 3g | sodium: 575mg

Peach-Glazed Chicken Drumsticks

Prep time: 10 minutes | Cook time: 20 minutes | Serves 4

8 chicken drumsticks (2-pound / 907-g), skin removed
Nonstick cooking spray
1 (15-ounce / 425-g) can sliced peaches in 100% juice, drained
¼ cup honey
¼ cup cider vinegar
3 garlic cloves
½ teaspoon smoked paprika
¼ teaspoon kosher or sea salt
¼ teaspoon freshly ground black pepper

1. Remove the chicken from the refrigerator.
2. Set one oven rack about 4 inches below the broiler element. Preheat the oven to 500°F (260°C). Line a large, rimmed baking sheet with aluminum foil. Place a wire cooling rack on the aluminum foil, and spray the rack with nonstick cooking spray. Set aside.
3. In a blender, combine the peaches, honey, vinegar, garlic, smoked paprika, salt, and pepper. Purée the ingredients until smooth.
4. Add the purée to a medium saucepan and bring to a boil over medium-high heat. Cook for 2 minutes, stirring constantly. Divide the sauce among two small bowls. The first bowl will be brushed on the chicken; set aside the second bowl for serving at the table.
5. Brush all sides of the chicken with about half the sauce (keeping half the sauce for a second coating), and place the drumsticks on the prepared rack. Roast for 10 minutes.
6. Remove the chicken from the oven and turn to the high broiler setting. Brush the chicken with the remaining sauce from the first bowl. Return the chicken to the oven and broil for 5 minutes. Turn the chicken; broil for 3 to 5 more minutes, until the internal temperature measures 165°F (74°C) on a meat thermometer, or until the juices run clear. Serve with the reserved sauce.

Per Serving
calories: 526 | fat: 22g | protein: 44g
carbs: 38g | fiber: 1g | sodium: 412mg

Parsley-Dijon Chicken and Potatoes

Prep time: 5 minutes | Cook time: 22 minutes | Serves 6

1 tablespoon extra-virgin olive oil
1½ pounds (680 g) boneless, skinless chicken thighs, cut into 1-inch cubes, patted dry
1½ pounds (680 g) Yukon Gold potatoes, unpeeled, cut into ½-inch cubes
2 garlic cloves, minced
¼ cup dry white wine
1 cup low-sodium
or no-salt-added chicken broth
1 tablespoon Dijon mustard
¼ teaspoon freshly ground black pepper
¼ teaspoon kosher or sea salt
1 cup chopped fresh flat-leaf (Italian) parsley, including stems
1 tablespoon freshly squeezed lemon juice

1. In a large skillet over medium-high heat, heat the oil. Add the chicken and cook for 5 minutes, stirring only after the chicken has browned on one side. Remove the chicken and reserve on a plate.
2. Add the potatoes to the skillet and cook for 5 minutes, stirring only after the potatoes have become golden and crispy on one side. Push the potatoes to the side of the skillet, add the garlic, and cook, stirring constantly, for 1 minute. Add the wine and cook for 1 minute, until nearly evaporated. Add the chicken broth, mustard, salt, pepper, and reserved chicken. Turn the heat to high and bring to a boil.
3. Once boiling, cover, reduce the heat to medium-low, and cook for 10 to 12 minutes, until the potatoes are tender and the internal temperature of the chicken measures 165°F (74°C) on a meat thermometer and any juices run clear.
4. During the last minute of cooking, stir in the parsley. Remove from the heat, stir in the lemon juice, and serve.

Per Serving
calories: 324 | fat: 9g | protein: 16g
carbs: 45g | fiber: 5g | sodium: 560mg

Chicken Breast with Tomato and Basil

Prep time: 10 minutes | Cook time: 20 minutes | Serves 4

Nonstick cooking spray
1 pound (454 g) boneless, skinless chicken breasts
2 tablespoons extra-virgin olive oil
¼ teaspoon freshly ground black pepper
¼ teaspoon kosher or sea salt
1 large tomato, sliced thinly
1 cup shredded Mozzarella or 4 ounces fresh Mozzarella cheese, diced
1 (14½-ounce / 411-g) can low-sodium or no-salt-added crushed tomatoes
2 tablespoons fresh torn basil leaves
4 teaspoons balsamic vinegar

1. Set one oven rack about 4 inches below the broiler element. Preheat the oven to 450ºF (235ºC). Line a large, rimmed baking sheet with aluminum foil. Place a wire cooling rack on the aluminum foil, and spray the rack with nonstick cooking spray. Set aside.
2. Cut the chicken into 4 pieces (if they aren't already). Put the chicken breasts in a large zip-top plastic bag. With a rolling pin or meat mallet, pound the chicken so it is evenly flattened, about ¼-inch thick. Add the oil, pepper, and salt to the bag. Reseal the bag, and massage the ingredients into the chicken. Take the chicken out of the bag and place it on the prepared wire rack.
3. Cook the chicken for 15 to 18 minutes, or until the internal temperature of the chicken is 165ºF (74ºC) on a meat thermometer and the juices run clear. Turn the oven to the high broiler setting. Layer the tomato slices on each chicken breast, and top with the Mozzarella. Broil the chicken for another 2 to 3 minutes, or until the cheese is melted (don't let the chicken burn on the edges). Remove the chicken from the oven.
4. While the chicken is cooking, pour the crushed tomatoes into a small, microwave-safe bowl. Cover the bowl with a paper towel, and microwave for about 1 minute on high, until hot. When you're ready to serve, divide the tomatoes among four dinner plates.

Place each chicken breast on top of the tomatoes. Top with the basil and a drizzle of balsamic vinegar.

Per Serving
calories: 258 | fat: 9g | protein: 14g
carbs: 28g | fiber: 3g | sodium: 573mg

Lemon-Garlic Whole Chicken and Potatoes

Prep time: 10 minutes | Cook time: 45 minutes | Serves 4 to 6

1 cup garlic, minced
1½ cups lemon juice
1 cup plus 2 tablespoons extra-virgin olive oil, divided
1½ teaspoons salt, divided
1 teaspoon freshly ground black pepper
1 whole chicken, cut into 8 pieces
1 pound (454 g) fingerling or red potatoes

1. Preheat the oven to 400ºF (205ºC).
2. In a large bowl, whisk together the garlic, lemon juice, 1 cup of olive oil, 1 teaspoon of salt, and pepper.
3. Put the chicken in a large baking dish and pour half of the lemon sauce over the chicken. Cover the baking dish with foil, and cook for 20 minutes.
4. Cut the potatoes in half, and toss to coat with 2 tablespoons olive oil and 1 teaspoon of salt. Put them on a baking sheet and bake for 20 minutes in the same oven as the chicken.
5. Take both the chicken and potatoes out of the oven. Using a spatula, transfer the potatoes to the baking dish with the chicken. Pour the remaining sauce over the potatoes and chicken. Bake for another 25 minutes.
6. Transfer the chicken and potatoes to a serving dish and spoon the garlic-lemon sauce from the pan on top.

Per Serving
calories: 959 | fat: 78g | protein: 33g
carbs: 37g | fiber: 4g | sodium: 1005mg

Stuffed Chicken Breast with Caprese

Prep time: 10 minutes | Cook time: 30 minutes | Serves 4

8 tablespoons extra-virgin olive oil, divided
2 (6-ounce / 170 g) boneless, skinless chicken breasts
4 ounces (113 g) frozen spinach, thawed and drained well
1 cup shredded fresh Mozzarella cheese
¼ cup chopped fresh basil
2 tablespoons chopped sun-dried tomatoes (preferably marinated in oil)
1 teaspoon salt, divided
1 teaspoon freshly ground black pepper, divided
½ teaspoon garlic powder
1 tablespoon balsamic vinegar

1. Preheat the oven to 375ºF (190ºC).
2. Drizzle 1 tablespoon olive oil in a small deep baking dish and swirl to coat the bottom.
3. Make a deep incision about 3- to 4-inches long along the length of each chicken breast to create a pocket. Using your knife or fingers, carefully increase the size of the pocket without cutting through the chicken breast. (Each breast will look like a change purse with an opening at the top.)
4. In a medium bowl, combine the spinach, Mozzarella, basil, sun-dried tomatoes, 2 tablespoons olive oil, ½ teaspoon salt, ½ teaspoon pepper, and the garlic powder and combine well with a fork.
5. Stuff half of the filling mixture into the pocket of each chicken breast, stuffing down to fully fill the pocket. Press the opening together with your fingers. You can use a couple toothpicks to pin it closed if you wish.
6. In a medium skillet, heat 2 tablespoons olive oil over medium-high heat. Carefully sear the chicken breasts until browned, 3 to 4 minutes per side, being careful to not let too much filling escape. Transfer to the prepared baking dish, incision-side up. Scrape up any filling that fell out in the skillet and add it to baking dish. Cover the pan with foil and bake until the chicken is cooked through, 30 to 40 minutes, depending on the thickness of the breasts.
7. Remove from the oven and rest, covered, for 10 minutes. Meanwhile, in a small bowl, whisk together the remaining 3 tablespoons olive oil, balsamic vinegar, ½ teaspoon salt, and ½ teaspoon pepper.
8. To serve, cut each chicken breast in half, widthwise, and serve a half chicken breast drizzled with oil and vinegar.

Per Serving
calories: 434 | fat: 34g | protein: 27g
carbs: 2g | fiber: 1g | sodium: 742mg

Chicken Shish Tawook

Prep time: 15 minutes | Cook time: 15 minutes | Serves 4 to 6

2 tablespoons garlic, minced
2 tablespoons tomato paste
1 teaspoon smoked paprika
½ cup lemon juice
½ cup extra-virgin olive oil
1½ teaspoons salt
½ teaspoon freshly ground black pepper
2 pounds (907 g) boneless and skinless chicken (breasts or thighs)
Rice, tzatziki, or hummus, for serving (optional)

1. In a large bowl, add the garlic, tomato paste, paprika, lemon juice, olive oil, salt, and pepper and whisk to combine.
2. Cut the chicken into ½-inch cubes and put them into the bowl; toss to coat with the marinade. Set aside for at least 10 minutes.
3. To grill, preheat the grill on high. Thread the chicken onto skewers and cook for 3 minutes per side, for a total of 9 minutes.
4. To cook in a pan, preheat the pan on high heat, add the chicken, and cook for 9 minutes, turning over the chicken using tongs.
5. Serve the chicken with rice, tzatziki, or hummus, if desired.

Per Serving
calories: 482 | fat: 32g | protein: 47g
carbs: 6g | fiber: 1g | sodium: 1298mg

Almond-Crusted Chicken Tenders with Honey

Prep time: 10 minutes | Cook time: 20 minutes | Serves 4

1 tablespoon honey
1 tablespoon whole-grain or Dijon mustard
¼ teaspoon freshly ground black pepper
¼ teaspoon kosher or sea salt
1 pound (454 g) boneless, skinless chicken breast tenders or tenderloins
1 cup almonds, roughly chopped
Nonstick cooking spray

1. Preheat the oven to 425°F (220°C). Line a large, rimmed baking sheet with parchment paper. Place a wire cooling rack on the parchment-lined baking sheet, and spray the rack well with nonstick cooking spray.
2. In a large bowl, combine the honey, mustard, pepper, and salt. Add the chicken and toss gently to coat. Set aside.
3. Dump the almonds onto a large sheet of parchment paper and spread them out. Press the coated chicken tenders into the nuts until evenly coated on all sides. Place the chicken on the prepared wire rack.
4. Bake in the preheated oven for 15 to 20 minutes, or until the internal temperature of the chicken measures 165°F (74°C) on a meat thermometer and any juices run clear.
5. Cool for 5 minutes before serving.

Per Serving
calories: 222 | fat: 7g | protein: 11g
carbs: 29g | fiber: 2g | sodium: 448mg

Traditional Chicken Shawarma

Prep time: 15 minutes | Cook time: 15 minutes | Serves 4 to 6

2 pounds (907 g) boneless and skinless chicken
½ cup lemon juice
½ cup extra-virgin olive oil
3 tablespoons minced garlic
1½ teaspoons salt
½ teaspoon freshly ground black pepper
½ teaspoon ground cardamom
½ teaspoon cinnamon
Hummus and pita bread, for serving (optional)

1. Cut the chicken into ¼-inch strips and put them into a large bowl.
2. In a separate bowl, whisk together the lemon juice, olive oil, garlic, salt, pepper, cardamom, and cinnamon.
3. Pour the dressing over the chicken and stir to coat all of the chicken.
4. Let the chicken sit for about 10 minutes.
5. Heat a large pan over medium-high heat and cook the chicken pieces for 12 minutes, using tongs to turn the chicken over every few minutes.
6. Serve with hummus and pita bread, if desired.

Per Serving
calories: 477 | fat: 32g | protein: 47g
carbs: 5g | fiber: 1g | sodium: 1234mg

Moroccan Chicken Meatballs

Prep time: 10 minutes | Cook time: 10 minutes | Serves 4 to 6

2 large shallots, diced
2 tablespoons finely chopped parsley
2 teaspoons paprika
1 teaspoon ground cumin
½ teaspoon ground coriander
½ teaspoon garlic powder
½ teaspoon salt
½ teaspoon freshly ground black pepper
⅛ teaspoon ground cardamom
1 pound (454 g) ground chicken
½ cup all-purpose flour, to coat
¼ cup olive oil, divided

1. In a bowl, combine the shallots, parsley, paprika, cumin, coriander, garlic powder, salt, pepper, and cardamom. Mix well.
2. Add the chicken to the spice mixture and mix well. Form into 1-inch balls flattened to about ½-inch thickness.
3. Put the flour in a bowl for dredging. Dip the balls into the flour until coated.
4. Pour enough oil to cover the bottom of a sauté pan or skillet and heat over medium heat. Working in batches, cook the meatballs, turning frequently, for 2 to 3 minutes on each side, until they are cooked through. Add more oil between batches as needed. Serve in a pita, topped with lettuce dressed with Creamy Yogurt Dressing.

Per Serving
calories: 405 | fat: 26g | protein: 24g
carbs: 20g | fiber: 1g | sodium: 387mg

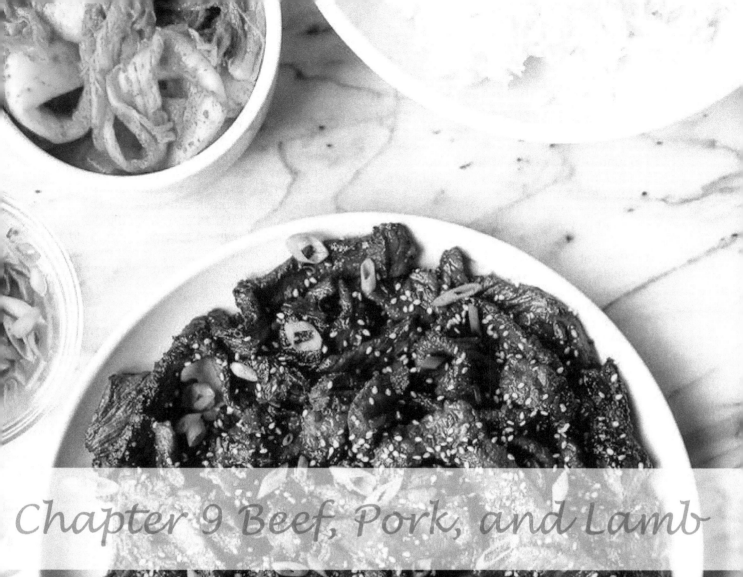
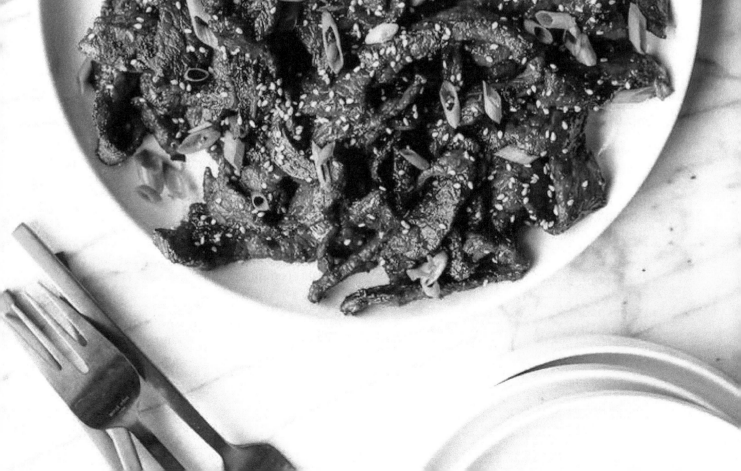

Chapter 9 Beef, Pork, and Lamb

Greek-Style Lamb Burgers

Prep time: 10 minutes | Cook time: 10 minutes | Serves 4

1 pound (454 g) ground lamb
½ teaspoon salt
½ teaspoon freshly ground black pepper

4 tablespoons feta cheese, crumbled
Buns, toppings, and tzatziki, for serving (optional)

1. Preheat a grill, grill pan, or lightly oiled skillet to high heat.
2. In a large bowl, using your hands, combine the lamb with the salt and pepper.
3. Divide the meat into 4 portions. Divide each portion in half to make a top and a bottom. Flatten each half into a 3-inch circle. Make a dent in the center of one of the halves and place 1 tablespoon of the feta cheese in the center. Place the second half of the patty on top of the feta cheese and press down to close the 2 halves together, making it resemble a round burger.
4. Cook the stuffed patty for 3 minutes on each side, for medium-well. Serve on a bun with your favorite toppings and tzatziki sauce, if desired.

Per Serving
calories: 345 | fat: 29g | protein: 20g
carbs: 1g | fiber: 0g | sodium: 462mg

Mediterranean Lamb Bowls

Prep time: 15 minutes | Cook time: 15 minutes | Serves 2

2 tablespoons extra-virgin olive oil
¼ cup diced yellow onion
1 pound (454 g) ground lamb
1 teaspoon dried mint
1 teaspoon dried parsley
½ teaspoon red pepper flakes
¼ teaspoon garlic powder

1 cup cooked rice
½ teaspoon za'atar seasoning
½ cup halved cherry tomatoes
1 cucumber, peeled and diced
1 cup store-bought hummus
1 cup crumbled feta cheese
2 pita breads, warmed (optional)

1. In a large sauté pan or skillet, heat the olive oil over medium heat and cook the onion for about 2 minutes, until fragrant. Add the lamb and mix well, breaking up the meat as you cook. Once the lamb is halfway cooked, add mint, parsley, red pepper flakes, and garlic powder.
2. In a medium bowl, mix together the cooked rice and za'atar, then divide between individual serving bowls. Add the seasoned lamb, then top the bowls with the tomatoes, cucumber, hummus, feta, and pita (if using).

Per Serving
calories: 1312 | fat: 96g | protein: 62g
carbs: 62g | fiber: 12g | sodium: 1454mg

Lemon-Rosemary Lamb Chops

Prep time: 10 minutes | Cook time: 10 minutes | Serves 6

4 large cloves garlic
1 cup lemon juice
⅓ cup fresh rosemary
1 cup extra-virgin olive oil

1½ teaspoons salt
1 teaspoon freshly ground black pepper
6 (1-inch-thick) lamb chops

1. In a food processor or blender, blend the garlic, lemon juice, rosemary, olive oil, salt, and black pepper for 15 seconds. Set aside.
2. Put the lamb chops in a large plastic zip-top bag or container. Cover the lamb with two-thirds of the rosemary dressing, making sure that all of the lamb chops are coated with the dressing. Let the lamb marinate in the fridge for 1 hour.
3. When you are almost ready to eat, take the lamb chops out of the fridge and let them sit on the counter-top for 20 minutes. Preheat a grill, grill pan, or lightly oiled skillet to high heat.
4. Cook the lamb chops for 3 minutes on each side. To serve, drizzle the lamb with the remaining dressing.

Per Serving
calories: 484 | fat: 42g | protein: 24g
carbs: 5g | fiber: 1g | sodium: 655mg

Braised Veal Shanks

Prep time: 10 minutes | Cook time: 2 hours | Serves 4

4 veal shanks, bone in
½ cup flour
4 tablespoons extra-virgin olive oil
1 large onion, chopped
5 cloves garlic, sliced
2 teaspoons salt
1 tablespoon fresh thyme
3 tablespoons tomato paste
6 cups water
Cooked noodles, for serving (optional)

1. Preheat the oven to 350ºF (180ºC).
2. Dredge the veal shanks in the flour.
3. Pour the olive oil into a large oven-safe pot or pan over medium heat; add the veal shanks. Brown the veal on both sides, about 4 minutes each side. Remove the veal from pot and set aside.
4. Add the onion, garlic, salt, thyme, and tomato paste to the pan and cook for 3 to 4 minutes. Add the water, and stir to combine.
5. Add the veal back to the pan, and bring to a simmer. Cover the pan with a lid or foil and bake for 1 hour and 50 minutes. Remove from the oven and serve with cooked noodles, if desired.

Per Serving
calories: 400 | fat: 19g | protein: 39g
carbs: 18g | fiber: 2g | sodium: 1368mg

Grilled Beef Kebabs

Prep time: 15 minutes | Cook time: 10 minutes | Serves 6

2 pounds (907 g) beef fillet
1½ teaspoons salt
1 teaspoon freshly ground black pepper
½ teaspoon ground allspice
½ teaspoon ground
nutmeg
⅓ cup extra-virgin olive oil
1 large onion, cut into 8 quarters
1 large red bell pepper, cut into 1-inch cubes

1. Preheat a grill, grill pan, or lightly oiled skillet to high heat.
2. Cut the beef into 1-inch cubes and put them in a large bowl.
3. In a small bowl, mix together the salt, black pepper, allspice, and nutmeg.
4. Pour the olive oil over the beef and toss to coat the beef. Then evenly sprinkle the seasoning over the beef and toss to coat all pieces.
5. Skewer the beef, alternating every 1 or 2 pieces with a piece of onion or bell pepper.
6. To cook, place the skewers on the grill or skillet, and turn every 2 to 3 minutes until all sides have cooked to desired doneness, 6 minutes for medium-rare, 8 minutes for well done. Serve warm.

Per Serving
calories: 485 | fat: 36g | protein: 35g
carbs: 4g | fiber: 1g | sodium: 1453mg

Mediterranean Grilled Skirt Steak

Prep time: 10 minutes | Cook time: 10 minutes | Serves 4

1 pound (454 g) skirt steak
1 teaspoon salt
½ teaspoon freshly ground black pepper
2 cups prepared hummus
1 tablespoon extra-virgin olive oil
½ cup pine nuts

1. Preheat a grill, grill pan, or lightly oiled skillet to medium heat.
2. Season both sides of the steak with salt and pepper.
3. Cook the meat on each side for 3 to 5 minutes; 3 minutes for medium, and 5 minutes on each side for well done. Let the meat rest for 5 minutes.
4. Slice the meat into thin strips.
5. Spread the hummus on a serving dish, and evenly distribute the beef on top of the hummus.
6. In a small saucepan, over low heat, add the olive oil and pine nuts. Toast them for 3 minutes, constantly stirring them with a spoon so that they don't burn.
7. Spoon the pine nuts over the beef and serve.

Per Serving
calories: 602 | fat: 41g | protein: 42g
carbs: 20g | fiber: 8g | sodium: 1141mg

Beef Kefta

Prep time: 10 minutes | Cook time: 5 minutes | Serves 4

1 medium onion	cumin
⅓ cup fresh Italian parsley	¼ teaspoon cinnamon
1 pound (454 g) ground beef	1 teaspoon salt
¼ teaspoon ground	½ teaspoon freshly ground black pepper

1. Preheat a grill or grill pan to high.
2. Mince the onion and parsley in a food processor until finely chopped.
3. In a large bowl, using your hands, combine the beef with the onion mix, ground cumin, cinnamon, salt, and pepper.
4. Divide the meat into 6 portions. Form each portion into a flat oval.
5. Place the patties on the grill or grill pan and cook for 3 minutes on each side.

Per Serving
calories: 203 | fat: 10g | protein: 24g
carbs: 3g | fiber: 1g | sodium: 655mg

Pork Souvlaki with Oregano

Prep time: 10 minutes | Cook time: 10 minutes | Serves 4

1 (1½-pound / 680-g) pork loin	1 tablespoon dried oregano
2 tablespoons garlic, minced	1 teaspoon salt
⅓ cup extra-virgin olive oil	Pita bread and tzatziki, for serving (optional)
⅓ cup lemon juice	

1. Cut the pork into 1-inch cubes and put them into a bowl or plastic zip-top bag.
2. In a large bowl, mix together the garlic, olive oil, lemon juice, oregano, and salt.
3. Pour the marinade over the pork and let it marinate for at least 1 hour.
4. Preheat a grill, grill pan, or lightly oiled skillet to high heat. Using wood or metal skewers, thread the pork onto the skewers.
5. Cook the skewers for 3 minutes on each side, for 12 minutes in total.
6. Serve with pita bread and tzatziki sauce, if desired.

Per Serving
calories: 416 | fat: 30g | protein: 32g
carbs: 5g | fiber: 1g | sodium: 1184mg

Beef and Potatoes with Tahini Sauce

Prep time: 10 minutes | Cook time: 30 minutes | Serves 4 to 6

2 POUNDS

1 pound (454 g) ground beef	potatoes
2 teaspoons salt, divided	2 tablespoons extra-virgin olive oil
½ teaspoon freshly ground black pepper	3 cups Greek yogurt
1 large onion, finely chopped	1 cup tahini
10 medium golden	3 cloves garlic, minced
	2 cups water

1. Preheat the oven to 450ºF (235ºC).
2. In a large bowl, using your hands, combine the beef with 1 teaspoon salt, black pepper, and the onion.
3. Form meatballs of medium size (about 1-inch), using about 2 tablespoons of the beef mixture. Place them in a deep 8-by-8-inch casserole dish.
4. Cut the potatoes into ¼-inch-thick slices. Toss them with the olive oil.
5. Lay the potato slices flat on a lined baking sheet.
6. Put the baking sheet with the potatoes and the casserole dish with the meatballs in the oven and bake for 20 minutes.
7. In a large bowl, mix together the yogurt, tahini, garlic, remaining 1 teaspoon salt, and water; set aside.
8. Once you take the meatballs and potatoes out of the oven, use a spatula to transfer the potatoes from the baking sheet to the casserole dish with the meatballs, and leave the beef drippings in the casserole dish for added flavor.
9. Reduce the oven temperature to 375ºF (190ºC) and pour the yogurt tahini sauce over the beef and potatoes. Return it to the oven for 10 minutes. Once baking is complete, serve warm with a side of rice or pita bread.

Per Serving
calories: 1078 | fat: 59g | protein: 58g
carbs: 89g | fiber: 11g | sodium: 1368mg

Filet Mignon with Mushroom-Red Wine Sauce

Prep time: 15 minutes | Cook time: 16 minutes | Serves 2

2 (3-ounce / 85-g) pieces filet mignon
2 tablespoons olive oil, divided
8 ounces (227 g) baby bella (cremini) mushrooms, quartered
⅓ cup large shallot, minced
2 teaspoons flour
2 teaspoons tomato paste
½ cup red wine
1 cup low-sodium
chicken stock
½ teaspoon dried thyme
1 sprig fresh rosemary
1 teaspoon herbes de Provence
¼ teaspoon salt
¼ teaspoon garlic powder
¼ teaspoon onion powder
Pinch freshly ground black pepper

1. Preheat the oven to 425°F (220°C) and set the oven rack to the middle position.
2. Remove the filets from the refrigerator about 30 minutes before you're ready to cook them. Pat them dry with a paper towel and let them rest while you prepare the mushroom sauce.
3. In a sauté pan, heat 1 tablespoon of olive oil over medium-high heat. Add the mushrooms and shallot and sauté for 10 minutes.
4. Add the flour and tomato paste and cook for another 30 seconds. Add the wine and scrape up any browned bits from the sauté pan. Add the chicken stock, thyme, and rosemary.
5. Stir the sauce so the flour doesn't form lumps and bring it to a boil. Once the sauce thickens, reduce the heat to the lowest setting and cover the pan to keep the sauce warm.
6. In a small bowl, combine the herbes de Provence, salt, garlic powder, onion powder, and pepper.
7. Rub the beef with the remaining 1 tablespoon of olive oil and season it on both sides with the herb mixture.
8. Heat an oven-safe sauté pan over medium-high heat. Add the beef and sear for 2½ minutes on each side. Then, transfer the pan to the oven for 5 more minutes to finish cooking. Use a meat

thermometer to check the internal temperature and remove it at 130°F for medium-rare.
9. Tent the meat with foil and let it rest for 5 minutes before serving topped with the mushroom sauce.

Per Serving
calories: 385 | fat: 20g | protein: 25g
carbs: 15g | fiber: 0g | sodium: 330mg

Honey Garlicky Pork Chops

Prep time: 10 minutes | Cook time: 16 minutes | Serves 4

4 pork chops, boneless or bone-in
¼ teaspoon salt
⅛ teaspoon freshly ground black pepper
3 tablespoons extra-virgin olive oil
5 tablespoons low-
sodium chicken broth, divided
6 garlic cloves, minced
¼ cup honey
2 tablespoons apple cider vinegar

1. Season the pork chops with salt and pepper and set aside.
2. In a large sauté pan or skillet, heat the oil over medium-high heat. Add the pork chops and sear for 5 minutes on each side, or until golden brown.
3. Once the searing is complete, move the pork to a dish and reduce the skillet heat from medium-high to medium. Add 3 tablespoons of chicken broth to the pan; this will loosen the bits and flavors from the bottom of the skillet.
4. Once the broth has evaporated, add the garlic to the skillet and cook for 15 to 20 seconds, until fragrant. Add the honey, vinegar, and the remaining 2 tablespoons of broth. Bring the heat back up to medium-high and continue to cook for 3 to 4 minutes.
5. Stir periodically; the sauce is ready once it's thickened slightly. Add the pork chops back into the pan, cover them with the sauce, and cook for 2 minutes. Serve.

Per Serving
calories: 302 | fat: 16g | protein: 22g
carbs: 19g | fiber: 0g | sodium: 753mg

Lamb Koftas with Lime Yogurt Sauce

Prep time: 30 minutes | Cook time: 15 minutes | Serves 4

1 pound (454 g) ground lamb
½ cup finely chopped fresh mint, plus 2 tablespoons
¼ cup almond or coconut flour
¼ cup finely chopped red onion
¼ cup toasted pine nuts
2 teaspoons ground cumin
1½ teaspoons salt, divided
1 teaspoon ground cinnamon
1 teaspoon ground ginger
½ teaspoon ground nutmeg
½ teaspoon freshly ground black pepper
1 cup plain whole-milk Greek yogurt
2 tablespoons extra-virgin olive oil
Zest and juice of 1 lime

1. Heat the oven broiler to the low setting. You can also bake these at high heat (450 to 475ºF / 235 to 245ºC) if you happen to have a very hot broiler. Submerge four wooden skewers in water and let soak at least 10 minutes to prevent them from burning.
2. In a large bowl, combine the lamb, ½ cup mint, almond flour, red onion, pine nuts, cumin, 1 teaspoon salt, cinnamon, ginger, nutmeg, and pepper and, using your hands, incorporate all the ingredients together well.
3. Form the mixture into 12 egg-shaped patties and let sit for 10 minutes.
4. Remove the skewers from the water, thread 3 patties onto each skewer, and place on a broiling pan or wire rack on top of a baking sheet lined with aluminum foil. Broil on the top rack until golden and cooked through, 8 to 12 minutes, flipping once halfway through cooking.
5. While the meat cooks, in a small bowl, combine the yogurt, olive oil, remaining 2 tablespoons chopped mint, remaining ½ teaspoon salt, and lime zest and juice and whisk to combine well. Keep cool until ready to use.
6. Serve the skewers with yogurt sauce.

Per Serving
calories: 500 | fat: 42g | protein: 23g
carbs: 9g | fiber: 2g | sodium: 969mg

Lamb Burgers with Harissa Mayo

Prep time: 15 minutes | Cook time: 13 minutes | Serves 2

½ small onion, minced
1 garlic clove, minced
2 teaspoons minced fresh parsley
2 teaspoons minced fresh mint
¼ teaspoon salt
Pinch freshly ground black pepper
1 teaspoon cumin
1 teaspoon smoked paprika
¼ teaspoon coriander
8 ounces (227 g) lean ground lamb
2 tablespoons olive oil mayonnaise
½ teaspoon harissa paste, plus more or less to taste
2 hamburger buns or pitas, fresh greens, tomato slices (optional, for serving)

1. Preheat the grill to medium-high, 350ºF (180ºC) to 400ºF (205ºC) and oil the grill grate. Alternatively, you can cook these in a heavy pan (cast iron is best) on the stovetop.
2. In a large bowl, combine the onion, garlic, parsley, mint, salt, pepper, cumin, paprika, and coriander. Add the lamb and, using your hands, combine the meat with the spices so they are evenly distributed. Form meat mixture into 2 patties.
3. Grill the burgers for 4 minutes per side, or until the internal temperature registers 160ºF (71ºC) for medium.
4. If cooking on the stovetop, heat the pan to medium-high and oil the pan. Cook the burgers for 5 to 6 minutes per side, or until the internal temperature registers 160ºF (71ºC).
5. While the burgers are cooking, combine the mayonnaise and harissa in a small bowl.
6. Serve the burgers with the harissa mayonnaise and slices of tomato and fresh greens on a bun or pita—or skip the bun altogether.

Per Serving
calories: 381 | fat: 20g | protein: 22g
carbs: 27g | fiber: 2g | sodium: 653mg

Turkish Lamb Stew with Pistachios

Prep time: 20 minutes | Cook time: 14 minutes | Serves 6

1 pound (454 g) bone-in or boneless lamb leg steak, center cut
1 tablespoon extra-virgin olive oil
1 cup chopped onion
½ cup diced carrot
1 teaspoon ground cumin
½ teaspoon ground cinnamon
¼ teaspoon kosher or sea salt
4 garlic cloves, minced
2 tablespoons tomato paste
1 tablespoon chopped canned chipotle pepper in adobo sauce
2 cups water
½ cup chopped prunes
1 (15-ounce / 425-g) can chickpeas, drained and rinsed
2 tablespoons freshly squeezed lemon juice
¼ cup chopped unsalted pistachios
Cooked couscous or bulgur, for serving (optional)

1. Slice the meat into 1-inch cubes. Pat dry with a few paper towels.
2. In a large stockpot over medium-high heat, heat the oil. Add the lamb and any bone, and cook for 4 minutes, stirring only after allowing the meat to brown on one side. Using a slotted spoon, transfer the lamb from the pot to a plate. It will not yet be fully cooked. Don't clean out the stockpot.
3. Put the onion, carrot, cumin, cinnamon, and salt in the pot and cook for 6 minutes, stirring occasionally. Push the vegetables to the edge of the pot. Add the garlic and cook for 1 minute, stirring constantly. Add the tomato paste and chipotle pepper, and cook for 1 minute more, stirring constantly while blending and mashing the tomato paste into the vegetables.
4. Return the lamb to the pot along with the water and prunes. Turn up the heat to high, and bring to a boil. Reduce the heat to medium-low and cook for 5 to 7 minutes more, until the stew thickens slightly. Stir in the chickpeas and cook for 1 minute. Remove the stew from the heat, and stir in the lemon juice. Sprinkle the pistachios on top and serve over couscous, if desired.

Per Serving

calories: 284 | fat: 9g | protein: 23g
carbs: 32g | fiber: 5g | sodium: 291mg

Moroccan Cheesy Meatballs

Prep time: 10 minutes | Cook time: 16 minutes | Serves 4

¼ cup finely chopped onion
¼ cup raisins, coarsely chopped
1 teaspoon ground cumin
½ teaspoon ground cinnamon
¼ teaspoon smoked paprika
1 large egg
1 pound (454 g) ground beef (93% lean) or ground lamb
$1/_3$ cup panko bread crumbs
1 teaspoon extra-virgin olive oil
1 (28-ounce / 794-g) can low-sodium or no-salt-added crushed tomatoes
Chopped fresh mint, feta cheese, and/or fresh orange or lemon wedges, for serving (optional)

1. In a large bowl, combine the onion, raisins, cumin, cinnamon, smoked paprika, and egg. Add the ground beef and bread crumbs and mix gently with your hands. Divide the mixture into 20 even portions, then wet your hands and roll each portion into a ball. Wash your hands.
2. In a large skillet over medium-high heat, heat the oil. Add the meatballs and cook for 8 minutes, rolling around every minute or so with tongs or a fork to brown them on most sides. (They won't be cooked through.) Transfer the meatballs to a paper towel–lined plate. Drain the fat out of the pan, and carefully wipe out the hot pan with a paper towel.
3. Return the meatballs to the pan, and pour the tomatoes over the meatballs. Cover and cook on medium-high heat until the sauce begins to bubble. Lower the heat to medium, cover partially, and cook for 7 to 8 more minutes, until the meatballs are cooked through. Garnish with fresh mint, feta cheese, and/or a squeeze of citrus, if desired, and serve.

Per Serving

calories: 284 | fat: 17g | protein: 26g
carbs: 10g | fiber: 5g | sodium: 113mg

Beef Short Ribs with Red Wine

Prep time: 10 minutes | Cook time: 1¾ hours | Serves 4

1½ pounds (680 g) boneless beef short ribs (if using bone-in, use 3½ pounds / 1.6 kg)
1 teaspoon salt
½ teaspoon freshly ground black pepper
½ teaspoon garlic powder
¼ cup extra-virgin olive oil
1 cup dry red wine (such as cabernet sauvignon or merlot)
2 to 3 cups beef broth, divided
4 sprigs rosemary

1. Preheat the oven to 350ºF (180ºC).
2. Season the short ribs with salt, pepper, and garlic powder. Let sit for 10 minutes.
3. In a Dutch oven or oven-safe deep skillet, heat the olive oil over medium-high heat.
4. When the oil is very hot, add the short ribs and brown until dark in color, 2 to 3 minutes per side. Remove the meat from the oil and keep warm.
5. Add the red wine and 2 cups beef broth to the Dutch oven, whisk together, and bring to a boil. Reduce the heat to low and simmer until the liquid is reduced to about 2 cups, about 10 minutes.
6. Return the short ribs to the liquid, which should come about halfway up the meat, adding up to 1 cup of remaining broth if needed. Cover and braise until the meat is very tender, about 1½ to 2 hours.
7. Remove from the oven and let sit, covered, for 10 minutes before serving. Serve warm, drizzled with cooking liquid.

Per Serving
calories: 792 | fat: 76g | protein: 25g
carbs: 2g | fiber: 0g | sodium: 783mg

Pork Tenderloin with Dijon Apple Sauce

Prep time: 10 minutes | Cook time: 20 minutes | Serves 8

1½ tablespoons extra-virgin olive oil
1 (12-ounce / 340-g) pork tenderloin
¼ teaspoon kosher salt
¼ teaspoon freshly ground black pepper
¼ cup apple jelly
¼ cup apple juice
2 to 3 tablespoons Dijon mustard
½ tablespoon cornstarch
½ tablespoon cream

1. Preheat the oven to 325ºF (163ºC).
2. In a large sauté pan or skillet, heat the olive oil over medium heat.
3. Add the pork to the skillet, using tongs to turn and sear the pork on all sides. Once seared, sprinkle pork with salt and pepper, and set it on a small baking sheet.
4. In the same skillet, with the juices from the pork, mix the apple jelly, juice, and mustard into the pan juices. Heat thoroughly over low heat, stirring consistently for 5 minutes. Spoon over the pork.
5. Put the pork in the oven and roast for 15 to 17 minutes, or 20 minutes per pound. Every 10 to 15 minutes, baste the pork with the apple-mustard sauce.
6. Once the pork tenderloin is done, remove it from the oven and let it rest for 15 minutes. Then, cut it into 1-inch slices.
7. In a small pot, blend the cornstarch with cream. Heat over low heat. Add the pan juices into the pot, stirring for 2 minutes, until thickened. Serve the sauce over the pork.

Per Serving
calories: 146 | fat: 7g | protein: 13g
carbs: 8g | fiber: 0g | sodium: 192mg

Herbed Lamb Burgers

Prep time: 15 minutes | Cook time: 15 minutes | Serves 4

1 pound (454 g) ground lamb	mint
½ small red onion, grated	¼ teaspoon paprika
1 tablespoon dried parsley	¼ teaspoon kosher salt
1 teaspoon dried oregano	⅛ teaspoon freshly ground black pepper
1 teaspoon ground cumin	Extra-virgin olive oil
1 teaspoon garlic powder	4 pita breads, for serving (optional)
½ teaspoon dried	Tzatziki sauce, for serving (optional)
	Pickled onions, for serving (optional)

1. In a bowl, combine the lamb, onion, parsley, oregano, cumin, garlic powder, mint, paprika, salt, and pepper. Divide the meat into 4 small balls and work into smooth discs.
2. In a large sauté pan or skillet, heat a drizzle of olive oil over medium heat or brush a grill with oil and set it to medium. Cook the patties for 4 to 5 minutes on each side, until cooked through and juices run clear.
3. Enjoy lamb burgers in pitas, topped with tzatziki sauce and pickled onions (if using).

Per Serving
calories: 328 | fat: 27g | protein: 19g
carbs: 2g | fiber: 1g | sodium: 215mg

Moroccan Pot Roast

Prep time: 15 minutes | Cook time: 50 minutes | Serves 4

8 ounces (227 g) mushrooms, sliced	1 small eggplant, peeled and diced
4 tablespoons extra-virgin olive oil	1¼ cups low-sodium beef broth
3 small onions, cut into 2-inch pieces	½ cup halved apricots
2 tablespoons paprika	⅓ cup golden raisins
1½ tablespoons garam masala	3 pounds (1.4 kg) beef chuck roast
2 teaspoons salt	2 tablespoons honey
¼ teaspoon ground white pepper	1 tablespoon dried mint
2 tablespoons tomato paste	2 cups cooked brown rice

1. Set an electric pressure cooker to Sauté and put the mushrooms and oil in the cooker. Sauté for 5 minutes, then add the onions, paprika, garam masala, salt, and white pepper. Stir in the tomato paste and continue to sauté.
2. Add the eggplant and sauté for 5 more minutes, until softened. Pour in the broth. Add the apricots and raisins. Sear the meat for 2 minutes on each side.
3. Close and lock the lid and set the pressure cooker to high for 50 minutes.
4. When cooking is complete, quick release the pressure. Carefully remove the lid, then remove the meat from the sauce and break it into pieces. While the meat is removed, stir honey and mint into the sauce.
5. Assemble plates with ½ cup of brown rice, ½ cup of pot roast sauce, and 3 to 5 pieces of pot roast.

Per Serving
calories: 829 | fat: 34g | protein: 69g
carbs: 70g | fiber: 11g | sodium: 1556mg

Braised Garlic Flank Steak with Artichokes

Prep time: 15 minutes | Cook time: 60 minutes | Serves 4 to 6

4 tablespoons grapeseed oil, divided
2 pounds (907 g) flank steak
1 (14-ounce / 397-g) can artichoke hearts, drained and roughly chopped
1 onion, diced
8 garlic cloves, chopped
1 (32-ounce / 907-g) container low-sodium beef broth
1 (14½-ounce / 411-g) can diced tomatoes, drained
1 cup tomato sauce
2 tablespoons tomato paste
1 teaspoon dried oregano
1 teaspoon dried parsley
1 teaspoon dried basil
½ teaspoon ground cumin
3 bay leaves
2 to 3 cups cooked couscous (optional)

1. Preheat the oven to 450ºF (235ºC).
2. In an oven-safe sauté pan or skillet, heat 3 tablespoons of oil on medium heat. Sear the steak for 2 minutes per side on both sides. Transfer the steak to the oven for 30 minutes, or until desired tenderness.
3. Meanwhile, in a large pot, combine the remaining 1 tablespoon of oil, artichoke hearts, onion, and garlic. Pour in the beef broth, tomatoes, tomato sauce, and tomato paste. Stir in oregano, parsley, basil, cumin, and bay leaves.
4. Cook the vegetables, covered, for 30 minutes. Remove bay leaf and serve with flank steak and ½ cup of couscous per plate, if using.

Per Serving
calories: 577 | fat: 28g | protein: 55g | carbs: 22g | fiber: 6g | sodium: 1405mg

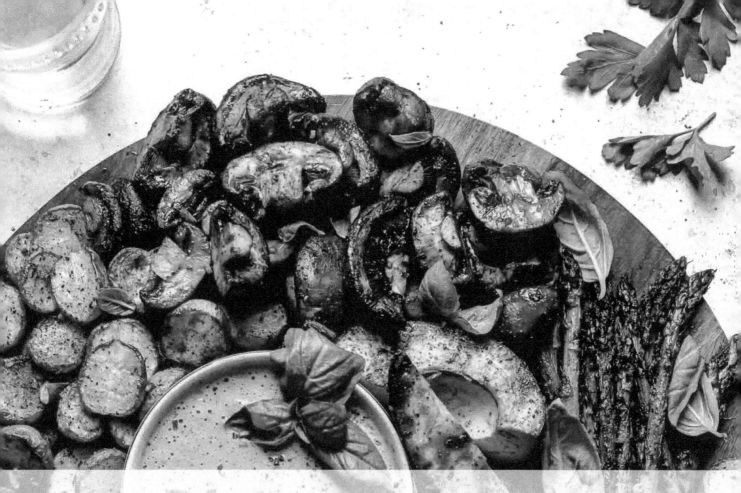
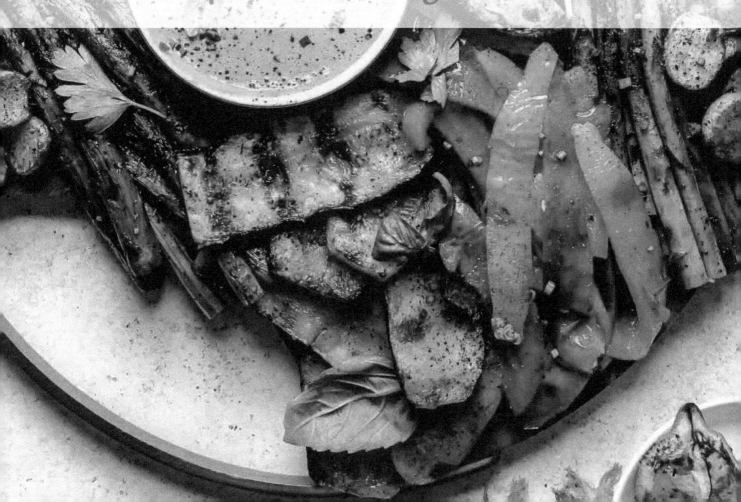

Chapter 10 Vegetables

Roasted Acorn Squash with Sage

Prep time: 10 minutes | Cook time: 35 minutes | Serves 6

2 acorn squash, medium to large
2 tablespoons extra-virgin olive oil
1 teaspoon salt, plus more for seasoning
5 tablespoons unsalted butter

(optional)
¼ cup chopped sage leaves
2 tablespoons fresh thyme leaves
½ teaspoon freshly ground black pepper

1. Preheat the oven to 400ºF (205ºC).
2. Cut the acorn squash in half lengthwise. Scrape out the seeds with a spoon and cut it horizontally into ¾-inch-thick slices.
3. In a large bowl, drizzle the squash with the olive oil, sprinkle with salt, and toss together to coat.
4. Lay the acorn squash flat on a baking sheet.
5. Put the baking sheet in the oven and bake the squash for 20 minutes. Flip squash over with a spatula and bake for another 15 minutes.
6. Melt the butter in a medium saucepan over medium heat.
7. Add the sage and thyme to the melted butter and let them cook for 30 seconds.
8. Transfer the cooked squash slices to a plate. Spoon the butter/herb mixture over the squash. Season with salt and black pepper. Serve warm.

Per Serving
calories: 188 | fat: 15g | protein: 1g
carbs: 16g | fiber: 3g | sodium: 393mg

Carrot and Bean Stuffed Peppers

Prep time: 20 minutes | Cook time: 30 minutes | Serves 6

6 large bell peppers, different colors
3 tablespoons extra-virgin olive oil
1 large onion, chopped
3 cloves garlic, minced

1 carrot, chopped
1 (16-ounce / 454-g) can garbanzo beans, rinsed and drained
3 cups cooked rice
1½ teaspoons salt
½ teaspoon freshly ground black pepper

1. Preheat the oven to 350ºF (180ºC).
2. Make sure to choose peppers that can stand upright. Cut off the pepper cap and remove the seeds, reserving the cap for later. Stand the peppers in a baking dish.
3. In a large skillet over medium heat, cook the olive oil, onion, garlic, and carrots for 3 minutes.
4. Stir in the garbanzo beans. Cook for another 3 minutes.
5. Remove the pan from the heat and spoon the cooked ingredients to a large bowl.
6. Add the rice, salt, and pepper; toss to combine.
7. Stuff each pepper to the top and then put the pepper caps back on.
8. Cover the baking dish with aluminum foil and bake for 25 minutes.
9. Remove the foil and bake for another 5 minutes.
10. Serve warm.

Per Serving
calories: 301 | fat: 9g | protein: 8g
carbs: 50g | fiber: 8g | sodium: 597mg

Rosemary Roasted Red Potatoes

Prep time: 5 minutes | Cook time: 20 minutes | Serves 6

1 pound (454 g) red potatoes, quartered
¼ cup olive oil
½ teaspoon kosher salt

¼ teaspoon black pepper
1 garlic clove, minced
4 rosemary sprigs

1. Preheat the air fryer to 360ºF (182ºC).
2. In a large bowl, toss the potatoes with the olive oil, salt, pepper, and garlic until well coated.
3. Pour the potatoes into the air fryer basket and top with the sprigs of rosemary.
4. Roast for 10 minutes, then stir or toss the potatoes and roast for 10 minutes more.
5. Remove the rosemary sprigs and serve the potatoes. Season with additional salt and pepper, if needed.

Per Serving
calories: 133 | fat: 9g | protein: 1g
carbs: 12g | fiber: 1g | sodium: 199mg

Easy Roasted Radishes

Prep time: 5 minutes | Cook time: 18 minutes | Serves 4

1 pound (454 g) radishes, ends trimmed if needed

2 tablespoons olive oil
½ teaspoon sea salt

1. Preheat the air fryer to 360ºF (182ºC).
2. In a large bowl, combine the radishes with olive oil and sea salt.
3. Pour the radishes into the air fryer and cook for 10 minutes. Stir or turn the radishes over and cook for 8 minutes more, then serve.

Per Serving
calories: 78 | fat: 9g | protein: 1g
carbs: 4g | fiber: 2g | sodium: 335mg

Zucchini with Garlic and Red Pepper

Prep time: 5 minutes | Cook time: 15 minutes | Serves 6

2 medium zucchini, cubed
1 red bell pepper, diced

2 garlic cloves, sliced
2 tablespoons olive oil
½ teaspoon salt

1. Preheat the air fryer to 380ºF (193ºC).
2. In a large bowl, mix together the zucchini, bell pepper, and garlic with the olive oil and salt.
3. Pour the mixture into the air fryer basket, and roast for 7 minutes. Shake or stir, then roast for 7 to 8 minutes more.

Per Serving
calories: 60 | fat: 5g | protein: 1g
carbs: 4g | fiber: 1g | sodium: 195mg

Savory Sweet Potatoes with Parmesan

Prep time: 10 minutes | Cook time: 18 minutes | Serves 4

2 large sweet potatoes, peeled and cubed
¼ cup olive oil
1 teaspoon dried

rosemary
½ teaspoon salt
2 tablespoons shredded Parmesan

1. Preheat the air fryer to 360ºF (182ºC).
2. In a large bowl, toss the sweet potatoes with the olive oil, rosemary, and salt.
3. Pour the potatoes into the air fryer basket and roast for 10 minutes, then stir the potatoes and sprinkle the Parmesan over the top. Continue roasting for 8 minutes more.
4. Serve hot and enjoy.

Per Serving
calories: 186 | fat: 14g | protein: 2g
carbs: 13g | fiber: 2g | sodium: 369mg

Ratatouille

Prep time: 15 minutes | Cook time: 40 minutes | Serves 6

2 russet potatoes, cubed
½ cup Roma tomatoes, cubed
1 eggplant, cubed
1 zucchini, cubed
1 red onion, chopped
1 red bell pepper, chopped
2 garlic cloves, minced
1 teaspoon dried mint
1 teaspoon dried

parsley
1 teaspoon dried oregano
½ teaspoon salt
½ teaspoon black pepper
¼ teaspoon red pepper flakes
⅓ cup olive oil
1 (8-ounce / 227-g) can tomato paste
¼ cup vegetable broth
¼ cup water

1. Preheat the air fryer to 320ºF (160ºC).
2. In a large bowl, combine the potatoes, tomatoes, eggplant, zucchini, onion, bell pepper, garlic, mint, parsley, oregano, salt, black pepper, and red pepper flakes.
3. In a small bowl, mix together the olive oil, tomato paste, broth, and water.
4. Pour the oil-and-tomato-paste mixture over the vegetables and toss until everything is coated.
5. Pour the coated vegetables into the air fryer basket in an even layer and roast for 20 minutes. After 20 minutes, stir well and spread out again. Roast for an additional 10 minutes, then repeat the process and cook for another 10 minutes.

Per Serving
calories: 280 | fat: 13g | protein: 6g
carbs: 40g | fiber: 7g | sodium: 264mg

Orange Roasted Brussels Sprouts

Prep time: 5 minutes | Cook time: 10 minutes | Serves 4

1 pound (454 g) Brussels sprouts, quartered
2 garlic cloves, minced

2 tablespoons olive oil
½ teaspoon salt
1 orange, cut into rings

1. Preheat the air fryer to 360ºF (182ºC).
2. In a large bowl, toss the quartered Brussels sprouts with the garlic, olive oil, and salt until well coated.
3. Pour the Brussels sprouts into the air fryer, lay the orange slices on top of them, and roast for 10 minutes.
4. Remove from the air fryer and set the orange slices aside. Toss the Brussels sprouts before serving.

Per Serving
calories: 111 | fat: 7g | protein: 4g
carbs: 11g | fiber: 4g | sodium: 319mg

Walnut Carrots with Honey Glaze

Prep time: 5 minutes | Cook time: 12 minutes | Serves 6

1 pound (454 g) baby carrots
2 tablespoons olive oil
¼ cup raw honey

¼ teaspoon ground cinnamon
¼ cup black walnuts, chopped

1. Preheat the air fryer to 360ºF (182ºC).
2. In a large bowl, toss the baby carrots with olive oil, honey, and cinnamon until well coated.
3. Pour into the air fryer and roast for 6 minutes. Shake the basket, sprinkle the walnuts on top, and roast for 6 minutes more.
4. Remove the carrots from the air fryer and serve.

Per Serving
calories: 146 | fat: 8g | protein: 1g
carbs: 20g | fiber: 3g | sodium: 60mg

Crispy Artichokes with Lemon

Prep time: 10 minutes | Cook time: 15 minutes | Serves 2

1 (15-ounce / 425-g) can artichoke hearts in water, drained
1 egg
1 tablespoon water

¼ cup whole wheat bread crumbs
¼ teaspoon salt
¼ teaspoon paprika
½ lemon

1. Preheat the air fryer to 380ºF (193ºC).
2. In a medium shallow bowl, beat together the egg and water until frothy.
3. In a separate medium shallow bowl, mix together the bread crumbs, salt, and paprika.
4. Dip each artichoke heart into the egg mixture, then into the bread crumb mixture, coating the outside with the crumbs. Place the artichokes hearts in a single layer of the air fryer basket.
5. Fry the artichoke hearts for 15 minutes.
6. Remove the artichokes from the air fryer, and squeeze fresh lemon juice over the top before serving.

Per Serving
calories: 91 | fat: 2g | protein: 5g
carbs: 16g | fiber: 8g | sodium: 505mg

Roasted Asparagus and Tomatoes

Prep time: 5 minutes | Cook time: 12 minutes | Serves 6

2 cups grape tomatoes
1 bunch asparagus, trimmed
2 tablespoons olive

oil
3 garlic cloves, minced
½ teaspoon kosher salt

1. Preheat the air fryer to 380ºF (193ºC).
2. In a large bowl, combine all of the ingredients, tossing until the vegetables are well coated with oil.
3. Pour the vegetable mixture into the air fryer basket and spread into a single layer, then roast for 12 minutes.

Per Serving
calories: 57 | fat: 5g | protein: 1g
carbs: 4g | fiber: 1g | sodium: 197mg

Lemon Green Beans with Red Onion

Prep time: 5 minutes | Cook time: 10 minutes | Serves 6

1 pound (454 g) fresh green beans, trimmed
½ red onion, sliced
2 tablespoons olive oil
½ teaspoon salt
¼ teaspoon black pepper
1 tablespoon lemon juice
Lemon wedges, for serving

1. Preheat the air fryer to 360ºF (182ºC). In a large bowl, toss the green beans, onion, olive oil, salt, pepper, and lemon juice until combined.
2. Pour the mixture into the air fryer and roast for 5 minutes. Stir well and roast for 5 minutes more.
3. Serve with lemon wedges.

Per Serving
calories: 67 | fat: 5g | protein: 1g
carbs: 6g | fiber: 2g | sodium: 199mg

Ricotta Stuffed Bell Peppers

Prep time: 10 minutes | Cook time: 20 minutes | Serves 4

2 red bell peppers
1 cup cooked brown rice
2 Roma tomatoes, diced
1 garlic clove, minced
¼ teaspoon salt
¼ teaspoon black pepper
4 ounces (113 g) ricotta
3 tablespoons fresh basil, chopped
3 tablespoons fresh oregano, chopped
¼ cup shredded Parmesan, for topping

1. Preheat the air fryer to 360ºF (182ºC).
2. Cut the bell peppers in half and remove the seeds and stem.
3. In a medium bowl, combine the brown rice, tomatoes, garlic, salt, and pepper.
4. Distribute the rice filling evenly among the four bell pepper halves.
5. In a small bowl, combine the ricotta, basil, and oregano. Put the herbed cheese over the top of the rice mixture in each bell pepper.
6. Place the bell peppers into the air fryer and roast for 20 minutes.

7. Remove and serve with shredded Parmesan on top.

Per Serving
calories: 156 | fat: 6g | protein: 8g
carbs: 19g | fiber: 3g | sodium: 264mg

Traditional Moussaka

Prep time: 20 minutes | Cook time: 40 minutes | Serves 6

2 large eggplants
2 teaspoons salt, divided
Olive oil spray, or olive oil for brushing
¼ cup extra-virgin olive oil
2 large onions, sliced
10 cloves garlic, sliced
2 (15-ounce / 425-g) cans diced tomatoes
1 (16-ounce / 454-g) can garbanzo beans, rinsed and drained
1 teaspoon dried oregano
½ teaspoon freshly ground black pepper

1. Slice the eggplant horizontally into ¼-inch-thick round disks. Sprinkle the eggplant slices with 1 teaspoon of salt and place in a colander for 30 minutes. This will draw out the excess water from the eggplant.
2. Preheat the oven to 450ºF (235ºC). Pat the slices of eggplant dry with a paper towel and spray each side with an olive oil spray or lightly brush each side with olive oil.
3. Arrange the eggplant in a single layer on a baking sheet. Put in the oven and bake for 10 minutes. Then, using a spatula, flip the slices over and bake for another 10 minutes.
4. In a large skillet add the olive oil, onions, garlic, and remaining 1 teaspoon of salt. Cook for 3 to 5 minutes stirring occasionally. Add the tomatoes, garbanzo beans, oregano, and black pepper. Simmer for 10 to 12 minutes, stirring occasionally.
5. Using a deep casserole dish, begin to layer, starting with eggplant, then the sauce. Repeat until all ingredients have been used. Bake in the oven for 20 minutes.
6. Remove from the oven and serve warm.

Per Serving
calories: 262 | fat: 11g | protein: 8g
carbs: 35g | fiber: 11g | sodium: 1043mg

Parmesan Stuffed Zucchini Boats

Prep time: 5 minutes | Cook time: 15 minutes | Serves 4

1 cup canned low-sodium chickpeas, drained and rinsed
1 cup no-sugar-added spaghetti

sauce
2 zucchinis
¼ cup shredded Parmesan cheese

1. Preheat the oven to 425ºF (220ºC).
2. In a medium bowl, stir together the chickpeas and spaghetti sauce.
3. Cut the zucchini in half lengthwise and scrape a spoon gently down the length of each half to remove the seeds.
4. Fill each zucchini half with the chickpea sauce and top with one-quarter of the Parmesan cheese.
5. Place the zucchini halves on a baking sheet and roast in the oven for 15 minutes.
6. Transfer to a plate. Let rest for 5 minutes before serving.

Per Serving
calories: 139 | fat: 4g | protein: 8g
carbs: 20g | fiber: 5g | sodium: 344mg

Spinach Cheese Pies

Prep time: 20 minutes | Cook time: 40 minutes | Serves 6 to 8

2 tablespoons extra-virgin olive oil
1 large onion, chopped
2 cloves garlic, minced

3 (1-pound / 454-g) bags of baby spinach, washed
1 cup feta cheese
1 large egg, beaten
Puff pastry sheets

1. Preheat the oven to 375ºF (190ºC).
2. In a large skillet over medium heat, cook the olive oil, onion, and garlic for 3 minutes.
3. Add the spinach to the skillet one bag at a time, letting it wilt in between each bag. Toss using tongs. Cook for 4 minutes. Once the spinach is cooked, drain any excess liquid from the pan.
4. In a large bowl, combine the feta cheese, egg, and cooked spinach.

5. Lay the puff pastry flat on a counter. Cut the pastry into 3-inch squares.
6. Place a tablespoon of the spinach mixture in the center of a puff-pastry square. Fold over one corner of the square to the diagonal corner, forming a triangle. Crimp the edges of the pie by pressing down with the tines of a fork to seal them together. Repeat until all squares are filled.
7. Place the pies on a parchment-lined baking sheet and bake for 25 to 30 minutes or until golden brown. Serve warm or at room temperature.

Per Serving
calories: 503 | fat: 32g | protein: 16g
carbs: 38g | fiber: 6g | sodium: 843mg

Vegetable Hummus Wraps

Prep time: 15 minutes | Cook time: 10 minutes | Serves 6

1 large eggplant
1 large onion
½ cup extra-virgin olive oil

1 teaspoon salt
6 lavash wraps or large pita bread
1 cup hummus

1. Preheat a grill, large grill pan, or lightly oiled large skillet on medium heat.
2. Slice the eggplant and onion into circles. Brush the vegetables with olive oil and sprinkle with salt.
3. Cook the vegetables on both sides, about 3 to 4 minutes each side.
4. To make the wrap, lay the lavash or pita flat. Spread about 2 tablespoons of hummus on the wrap.
5. Evenly divide the vegetables among the wraps, layering them along one side of the wrap. Gently fold over the side of the wrap with the vegetables, tucking them in and making a tight wrap.
6. Lay the wrap seam side-down and cut in half or thirds.
7. You can also wrap each sandwich with plastic wrap to help it hold its shape and eat it later.

Per Serving
calories: 362 | fat: 26g | protein: 15g
carbs: 28g | fiber: 11g | sodium: 1069mg

Parmesan Butternut Squash

Prep time: 15 minutes | Cook time: 20 minutes | Serves 4

2½ cups butternut squash, cubed into 1-inch pieces (approximately 1 medium)
2 tablespoons olive oil
¼ teaspoon salt
¼ teaspoon garlic powder
¼ teaspoon black pepper
1 tablespoon fresh thyme
¼ cup grated Parmesan

1. Preheat the air fryer to 360ºF (182ºC).
2. In a large bowl, combine the cubed squash with the olive oil, salt, garlic powder, pepper, and thyme until the squash is well coated.
3. Pour this mixture into the air fryer basket, and roast for 10 minutes. Stir and roast another 8 to 10 minutes more.
4. Remove the squash from the air fryer and toss with freshly grated Parmesan before serving.

Per Serving
calories: 127 | fat: 9g | protein: 3g
carbs: 11g | fiber: 2g | sodium: 262mg

Garlic Eggplant Slices

Prep time: 5 minutes | Cook time: 25 minutes | Serves 4

1 egg
1 tablespoon water
½ cup whole wheat bread crumbs
1 teaspoon garlic powder
½ teaspoon dried
oregano
½ teaspoon salt
½ teaspoon paprika
1 medium eggplant, sliced into ¼-inch-thick rounds
1 tablespoon olive oil

1. Preheat the air fryer to 360ºF (182ºC).
2. In a medium shallow bowl, beat together the egg and water until frothy.
3. In a separate medium shallow bowl, mix together bread crumbs, garlic powder, oregano, salt, and paprika.
4. Dip each eggplant slice into the egg mixture, then into the bread crumb mixture, coating the outside with crumbs. Place the slices in a single layer in the bottom of the air fryer basket.

5. Drizzle the tops of the eggplant slices with the olive oil, then fry for 15 minutes. Turn each slice and cook for an additional 10 minutes.

Per Serving
calories: 137 | fat: 5g | protein: 5g
carbs: 19g | fiber: 5g | sodium: 409mg

Cheesy Sweet Potato Burgers

Prep time: 10 minutes | Cook time: 19 to 20 minutes | Serves 4

1 large sweet potato (about 8 ounces / 227 g)
2 tablespoons extra-virgin olive oil, divided
1 cup chopped onion
1 large egg
1 garlic clove
1 cup old-fashioned
rolled oats
1 tablespoon dried oregano
1 tablespoon balsamic vinegar
¼ teaspoon kosher salt
½ cup crumbled Gorgonzola cheese

1. Using a fork, pierce the sweet potato all over and microwave on high for 4 to 5 minutes, until softened in the center. Cool slightly before slicing in half.
2. Meanwhile, in a large skillet over medium-high heat, heat 1 tablespoon of the olive oil. Add the onion and sauté for 5 minutes.
3. Spoon the sweet potato flesh out of the skin and put the flesh in a food processor. Add the cooked onion, egg, garlic, oats, oregano, vinegar and salt. Pulse until smooth. Add the cheese and pulse four times to barely combine.
4. Form the mixture into four burgers. Place the burgers on a plate, and press to flatten each to about ¾-inch thick.
5. Wipe out the skillet with a paper towel. Heat the remaining 1 tablespoon of the oil over medium-high heat for about 2 minutes. Add the burgers to the hot oil, then reduce the heat to medium. Cook the burgers for 5 minutes per side.
6. Transfer the burgers to a plate and serve.

Per Serving
calories: 290 | fat: 12g | protein: 12g
carbs: 43g | fiber: 8g | sodium: 566mg

Dill Beets

Prep time: 10 minutes | Cook time: 30 minutes | Serves 4

4 beets, cleaned, peeled, and sliced
1 garlic clove, minced
2 tablespoons chopped fresh dill
¼ teaspoon salt
¼ teaspoon black pepper
3 tablespoons olive oil

1. Preheat the air fryer to 380ºF (193ºC).
2. In a large bowl, mix together all of the ingredients so the beets are well coated with the oil.
3. Pour the beet mixture into the air fryer basket, and roast for 15 minutes before stirring, then continue roasting for 15 minutes more.

Per Serving
calories: 126 | fat: 10g | protein: 1g
carbs: 8g | fiber: 2g | sodium: 210mg

Mushrooms and Asparagus Farrotto

Prep time: 15 minutes | Cook time: 16 minutes | Serves 2

½ ounce (14 g) dried porcini mushrooms
1 cup hot water
3 cups low-sodium vegetable stock
2 tablespoons olive oil
½ large onion, minced
1 garlic clove
1 cup diced mushrooms
¾ cup farro
½ cup dry white wine
½ teaspoon dried thyme
4 ounces (113 g) asparagus, cut into ½-inch pieces
2 tablespoons grated Parmesan cheese
Salt, to taste

1. Soak the dried mushrooms in the hot water for about 15 minutes. When they're softened, drain the mushrooms, reserving the liquid. (I like to strain the liquid through a coffee filter in case there's any grit.) Mince the porcini mushrooms.
2. Add the mushroom liquid and vegetable stock to a medium saucepan and bring it to a boil. Reduce the heat to low just to keep it warm.
3. Heat the olive oil in a Dutch oven over high heat. Add the onion, garlic, and mushrooms, and sauté for 10 minutes.
4. Add the farro to the Dutch oven and sauté it for 3 minutes to toast.
5. Add the wine, thyme, and one ladleful of the hot mushroom and chicken stock. Bring it to a boil while stirring the farro. Do not cover the pot while the farro is cooking.
6. Reduce the heat to medium. When the liquid is absorbed, add another ladleful or two at a time to the pot, stirring occasionally, until the farro is cooked through. Keep an eye on the heat, to make sure it doesn't cook too quickly.
7. When the farro is al dente, add the asparagus and another ladleful of stock. Cook for another 3 to 5 minutes, or until the asparagus is softened.
8. Stir in Parmesan cheese and season with salt.

Per Serving
calories: 341 | fat: 15g | protein: 13g
carbs: 26g | fiber: 4g | sodium: 259mg

Butternut Noodles with Mushrooms

Prep time: 10 minutes | Cook time: 12 minutes | Serves 4

¼ cup extra-virgin olive oil
1 pound (454 g) cremini mushrooms, sliced
½ red onion, finely chopped
1 teaspoon dried thyme
½ teaspoon sea salt
3 garlic cloves, minced
½ cup dry white wine
Pinch of red pepper flakes
4 cups butternut noodles
4 ounces (113 g) grated Parmesan cheese

1. In a large skillet over medium-high heat, heat the olive oil until shimmering. Add the mushrooms, onion, thyme, and salt to the skillet. Cook for about 6 minutes, stirring occasionally, or until the mushrooms start to brown. Add the garlic and sauté for 30 seconds. Stir in the white wine and red pepper flakes.
2. Fold in the noodles. Cook for about 5 minutes, stirring occasionally, or until the noodles are tender.
3. Serve topped with the grated Parmesan.

Per Serving
calories: 244 | fat: 14g | protein: 4g
carbs: 22g | fiber: 4g | sodium: 159mg

Eggplant and Zucchini Gratin

Prep time: 10 minutes | Cook time: 19 minutes | Serves 6

2 large zucchini, finely chopped
1 large eggplant, finely chopped
¼ teaspoon kosher salt
¼ teaspoon freshly ground black pepper
3 tablespoons extra-virgin olive oil, divided
¾ cup unsweetened almond milk
1 tablespoon all-purpose flour
⅓ cup plus 2 tablespoons grated Parmesan cheese, divided
1 cup chopped tomato
1 cup diced fresh Mozzarella
¼ cup fresh basil leaves

1. Preheat the oven to 425ºF (220ºC).
2. In a large bowl, toss together the zucchini, eggplant, salt and pepper.
3. In a large skillet over medium-high heat, heat 1 tablespoon of the oil. Add half of the veggie mixture to the skillet. Stir a few times, then cover and cook for about 4 minutes, stirring occasionally. Pour the cooked veggies into a baking dish. Place the skillet back on the heat, add 1 tablespoon of the oil and repeat with the remaining veggies. Add the veggies to the baking dish.
4. Meanwhile, heat the milk in the microwave for 1 minute. Set aside.
5. Place a medium saucepan over medium heat. Add the remaining 1 tablespoon of the oil and flour to the saucepan. Whisk together until well blended.
6. Slowly pour the warm milk into the saucepan, whisking the entire time. Continue to whisk frequently until the mixture thickens a bit. Add ⅓ cup of the Parmesan cheese and whisk until melted. Pour the cheese sauce over the vegetables in the baking dish and mix well.
7. Fold in the tomatoes and Mozzarella cheese. Roast in the oven for 10 minutes, or until the gratin is almost set and not runny.
8. Top with the fresh basil leaves and the remaining 2 tablespoons of the Parmesan cheese before serving.

Per Serving
calories: 122 | fat: 5g | protein: 10g
carbs: 11g | fiber: 4g | sodium: 364mg

Veggie-Stuffed Portabello Mushrooms

Prep time: 5 minutes | Cook time: 24 to 25 minutes | Serves 6

3 tablespoons extra-virgin olive oil, divided
1 cup diced onion
2 garlic cloves, minced
1 large zucchini, diced
3 cups chopped mushrooms
1 cup chopped tomato
1 teaspoon dried
oregano
¼ teaspoon kosher salt
¼ teaspoon crushed red pepper
6 large portabello mushrooms, stems and gills removed
Cooking spray
4 ounces (113 g) fresh Mozzarella cheese, shredded

1. In a large skillet over medium heat, heat 2 tablespoons of the oil. Add the onion and sauté for 4 minutes. Stir in the garlic and sauté for 1 minute.
2. Stir in the zucchini, mushrooms, tomato, oregano, salt and red pepper. Cook for 10 minutes, stirring constantly. Remove from the heat.
3. Meanwhile, heat a grill pan over medium-high heat.
4. Brush the remaining 1 tablespoon of the oil over the portabello mushroom caps. Place the mushrooms, bottom-side down, on the grill pan. Cover with a sheet of aluminum foil sprayed with nonstick cooking spray. Cook for 5 minutes.
5. Flip the mushroom caps over, and spoon about ½ cup of the cooked vegetable mixture into each cap. Top each with about 2½ tablespoons of the Mozzarella.
6. Cover and grill for 4 to 5 minutes, or until the cheese is melted.
7. Using a spatula, transfer the portabello mushrooms to a plate. Let cool for about 5 minutes before serving.

Per Serving
calories: 111 | fat: 4g | protein: 11g
carbs: 11g | fiber: 4g | sodium: 314mg

Tabbouleh Stuffed Tomatoes

Prep time: 15 minutes | Cook time: 10 minutes | Serves 4

8 medium beefsteak or similar tomatoes
3 tablespoons extra-virgin olive oil, divided
½ cup water
½ cup uncooked regular or whole-wheat couscous
1½ cups minced fresh curly parsley
⅓ cup minced fresh
mint
2 scallions, green and white parts, chopped
¼ teaspoon freshly ground black pepper
¼ teaspoon kosher or sea salt
1 medium lemon
4 teaspoons honey
⅓ cup chopped almonds

1. Preheat the oven to 400ºF (205ºC).
2. Slice the top off each tomato and set aside. Scoop out all the flesh inside, and put the tops, flesh, and seeds in a large mixing bowl.
3. Grease a baking dish with 1 tablespoon of oil. Place the carved-out tomatoes in the baking dish, and cover with aluminum foil. Roast for 10 minutes.
4. While the tomatoes are cooking, make the couscous by bringing the water to boil in a medium saucepan. Pour in the couscous, remove from the heat, and cover. Let sit for 5 minutes, then stir with a fork.
5. While the couscous is cooking, chop up the tomato flesh and tops. Drain off the excess tomato water using a colander. Measure out 1 cup of the chopped tomatoes (reserve any remaining chopped tomatoes for another use). Add the cup of tomatoes back into the mixing bowl. Mix in the parsley, mint, scallions, pepper, and salt.
6. Using a Microplane or citrus grater, zest the lemon into the mixing bowl. Halve the lemon, and squeeze the juice through a strainer (to catch the seeds) from both halves into the bowl with the tomato mixture. Mix well.
7. When the couscous is ready, add it to the tomato mixture and mix well.
8. With oven mitts, carefully remove the tomatoes from the oven. Divide the tabbouleh evenly among the tomatoes and stuff them, using a spoon to press

the filling down so it all fits. Cover the pan with the foil and return it to the oven. Cook for another 8 to 10 minutes, or until the tomatoes are tender-firm. (If you prefer softer tomatoes, roast for an additional 10 minutes.) Before serving, top each tomato with a drizzle of ½ teaspoon of honey and about 2 teaspoons of almonds.

Per Serving
calories: 160 | fat: 6g | protein: 5g
carbs: 22g | fiber: 4g | sodium: 351mg

Garlicky Broccoli Rabe

Prep time: 10 minutes | Cook time: 5 to 6 minutes | Serves 4

14 ounces (397 g) broccoli rabe, trimmed and cut into 1-inch pieces
2 teaspoons salt, plus more for seasoning
Black pepper, to taste
2 tablespoons extra-virgin olive oil
3 garlic cloves, minced
¼ teaspoon red pepper flakes

1. Bring 3 quarts water to a boil in a large saucepan. Add the broccoli rabe and 2 teaspoons of the salt to the boiling water and cook for 2 to 3 minutes, or until wilted and tender.
2. Drain the broccoli rabe. Transfer to ice water and let sit until chilled. Drain again and pat dry.
3. In a skillet over medium heat, heat the oil and add the garlic and red pepper flakes. Sauté for about 2 minutes, or until the garlic begins to sizzle.
4. Increase the heat to medium-high. Stir in the broccoli rabe and cook for about 1 minute, or until heated through, stirring constantly. Season with salt and pepper.
5. Serve immediately.

Per Serving
calories: 87 | fat: 7g | protein: 3g
carbs: 4g | fiber: 3g | sodium: 1196mg

Beet and Watercress Salad

Prep time: 15 minutes | Cook time: 8 minutes | Serves 4

2 pounds (907 g) beets, scrubbed, trimmed and cut into ¾-inch pieces
½ cup water
1 teaspoon caraway seeds
½ teaspoon table salt, plus more for seasoning
1 cup plain Greek yogurt
1 small garlic clove, minced
5 ounces (142 g) watercress, torn into bite-size pieces
1 tablespoon extra-virgin olive oil, divided, plus more for drizzling
1 tablespoon white wine vinegar, divided
Black pepper, to taste
1 teaspoon grated orange zest
2 tablespoons orange juice
¼ cup coarsely chopped fresh dill
¼ cup hazelnuts, toasted, skinned and chopped
Coarse sea salt, to taste

1. Combine the beets, water, caraway seeds and table salt in the Instant Pot. Set the lid in place. Select the Manual mode and set the cooking time for 8 minutes on High Pressure. When the timer goes off, do a quick pressure release.
2. Carefully open the lid. Using a slotted spoon, transfer the beets to a plate. Set aside to cool slightly.
3. In a small bowl, combine the yogurt, garlic and 3 tablespoons of the beet cooking liquid. In a large bowl, toss the watercress with 2 teaspoons of the oil and 1 teaspoon of the vinegar. Season with table salt and pepper.
4. Spread the yogurt mixture over a serving dish. Arrange the watercress on top of the yogurt mixture, leaving 1-inch border of the yogurt mixture.
5. Add the beets to now-empty large bowl and toss with the orange zest and juice, the remaining 2 teaspoons of the vinegar and the remaining 1 teaspoon of the oil. Season with table salt and pepper.
6. Arrange the beets on top of the watercress mixture. Drizzle with the olive oil and sprinkle with the dill, hazelnuts and sea salt.
7. Serve immediately.

Per Serving
calories: 240 | fat: 15g | protein: 9g
carbs: 19g | fiber: 5g | sodium: 440mg

Zoodles with Walnut Pesto

Prep time: 10 minutes | Cook time: 10 minutes | Serves 4

4 medium zucchini, spiralized
¼ cup extra-virgin olive oil, divided
1 teaspoon minced garlic, divided
½ teaspoon crushed red pepper
¼ teaspoon freshly ground black pepper, divided
¼ teaspoon kosher salt, divided
2 tablespoons grated Parmesan cheese, divided
1 cup packed fresh basil leaves
¾ cup walnut pieces, divided

1. In a large bowl, stir together the zoodles, 1 tablespoon of the olive oil, ½ teaspoon of the minced garlic, red pepper, ⅛ teaspoon of the black pepper and ⅛ teaspoon of the salt. Set aside.
2. Heat ½ tablespoon of the oil in a large skillet over medium-high heat. Add half of the zoodles to the skillet and cook for 5 minutes, stirring constantly. Transfer the cooked zoodles into a bowl. Repeat with another ½ tablespoon of the oil and the remaining zoodles. When done, add the cooked zoodles to the bowl.
3. Make the pesto: In a food processor, combine the remaining ½ teaspoon of the minced garlic, ⅛ teaspoon of the black pepper and ⅛ teaspoon of the salt, 1 tablespoon of the Parmesan, basil leaves and ¼ cup of the walnuts. Pulse until smooth and then slowly drizzle the remaining 2 tablespoons of the oil into the pesto. Pulse again until well combined.
4. Add the pesto to the zoodles along with the remaining 1 tablespoon of the Parmesan and the remaining ½ cup of the walnuts. Toss to coat well.
5. Serve immediately.

Per Serving
calories: 166 | fat: 16g | protein: 4g
carbs: 3g | fiber: 2g | sodium: 307mg

Mini Potatoes Bake

Prep time: 10 minutes | Cook time: 30 minutes | Serves 2

10 ounces (283 g) golden mini potatoes, halved
4 tablespoons extra-virgin olive oil
2 teaspoons dried, minced garlic
1 teaspoon onion salt
½ teaspoon paprika
¼ teaspoon freshly ground black pepper
¼ teaspoon red pepper flakes
¼ teaspoon dried dill

1. Preheat the oven to 400ºF (205ºC).
2. Soak the potatoes and put in a bowl of ice water for 30 minutes. Change the water if you return and the water is milky.
3. Rinse and dry the potatoes, then put them on a baking sheet.
4. Drizzle the potatoes with oil and sprinkle with the garlic, onion salt, paprika, pepper, red pepper flakes, and dill. Using tongs or your hands, toss well to coat.
5. Lower the heat to 375ºF (190ºC), add potatoes to the oven, and bake for 20 minutes.
6. At 20 minutes, check and flip potatoes. Bake for another 10 minutes, or until the potatoes are fork-tender.

Per Serving (½ cup)
calories: 344 | fat: 27g | protein: 3g
carbs: 24g | fiber: 3g | sodium: 723mg

Sautéed Cabbage with Parsley

Prep time: 10 minutes | Cook time: 12 to 14 minutes | Serves 4 to 6

1 small head green cabbage (about 1¼ pounds / 567 g), cored and sliced thin
2 tablespoons extra-virgin olive oil, divided
1 onion, halved and sliced thin
¾ teaspoon salt, divided
¼ teaspoon black pepper
¼ cup chopped fresh parsley
1½ teaspoons lemon juice

1. Place the cabbage in a large bowl with cold water. Let sit for 3 minutes. Drain well.
2. Heat 1 tablespoon of the oil in a skillet over medium-high heat until shimmering.

Add the onion and ¼ teaspoon of the salt and cook for 5 to 7 minutes, or until softened and lightly browned. Transfer to a bowl.

3. Heat the remaining 1 tablespoon of the oil in now-empty skillet over medium-high heat until shimmering. Add the cabbage and sprinkle with the remaining ½ teaspoon of the salt and black pepper. Cover and cook for about 3 minutes, without stirring, or until cabbage is wilted and lightly browned on bottom.
4. Stir and continue to cook for about 4 minutes, uncovered, or until the cabbage is crisp-tender and lightly browned in places, stirring once halfway through cooking. Off heat, stir in the cooked onion, parsley and lemon juice.
5. Transfer to a plate and serve.

Per Serving
calories: 117 | fat: 7g | protein: 3g
carbs: 13g | fiber: 5g | sodium: 472mg

Orange-Honey Roasted Broccoli

Prep time: 5 minutes | Cook time: 12 minutes | Serves 6

4 cups broccoli florets (approximately 1 large head)
2 tablespoons olive oil
½ teaspoon salt
½ cup orange juice
1 tablespoon raw honey
Orange wedges, for serving (optional)

1. Preheat the air fryer to 360ºF (182ºC).
2. In a large bowl, combine the broccoli, olive oil, salt, orange juice, and honey. Toss the broccoli in the liquid until well coated.
3. Pour the broccoli mixture into the air fryer basket and cook for 6 minutes. Stir and cook for 6 minutes more.
4. Serve alone or with orange wedges for additional citrus flavor, if desired.

Per Serving
calories: 80 | fat: 5g | protein: 2g
carbs: 9g | fiber: 2g | sodium: 203mg

Braised Cauliflower with White Wine

Prep time: 10 minutes | Cook time: 12 to 16 minutes | Serves 4 to 6

3 tablespoons plus 1 teaspoon extra-virgin olive oil, divided
3 garlic cloves, minced
⅛ teaspoon red pepper flakes
1 head cauliflower (2 pounds / 907 g), cored and cut into
1½-inch florets
¼ teaspoon salt, plus more for seasoning
Black pepper, to taste
⅓ cup vegetable broth
⅓ cup dry white wine
2 tablespoons minced fresh parsley

1. Combine 1 teaspoon of the oil, garlic and pepper flakes in small bowl.
2. Heat the remaining 3 tablespoons of the oil in a skillet over medium-high heat until shimmering. Add the cauliflower and ¼ teaspoon of the salt and cook for 7 to 9 minutes, stirring occasionally, or until florets are golden brown.
3. Push the cauliflower to sides of the skillet. Add the garlic mixture to the center of the skillet. Cook for about 30 seconds, or until fragrant. Stir the garlic mixture into the cauliflower.
4. Pour in the broth and wine and bring to simmer. Reduce the heat to medium-low. Cover and cook for 4 to 6 minutes, or until the cauliflower is crisp-tender. Off heat, stir in the parsley and season with salt and pepper.
5. Serve immediately.

Per Serving
calories: 143 | fat: 11g | protein: 3g
carbs: 8g | fiber: 3g | sodium: 263mg

Cauliflower Steaks with Arugula

Prep time: 5 minutes | Cook time: 20 minutes | Serves 4

Cauliflower:
1 head cauliflower
Cooking spray
½ teaspoon garlic
powder
4 cups arugula

Dressing:
1½ tablespoons extra-virgin olive oil
1½ tablespoons
honey mustard
1 teaspoon freshly squeezed lemon juice

1. Preheat the oven to 425ºF (220ºC).
2. Remove the leaves from the cauliflower head, and cut it in half lengthwise. Cut 1½-inch-thick steaks from each half.
3. Spritz both sides of each steak with cooking spray and season both sides with the garlic powder.
4. Place the cauliflower steaks on a baking sheet, cover with foil, and roast in the oven for 10 minutes.
5. Remove the baking sheet from the oven and gently pull back the foil to avoid the steam. Flip the steaks, then roast uncovered for 10 minutes more.
6. Meanwhile, make the dressing: Whisk together the olive oil, honey mustard and lemon juice in a small bowl.
7. When the cauliflower steaks are done, divide into four equal portions. Top each portion with one-quarter of the arugula and dressing.
8. Serve immediately.

Per Serving
calories: 115 | fat: 6g | protein: 5g
carbs: 14g | fiber: 4g | sodium: 97mg

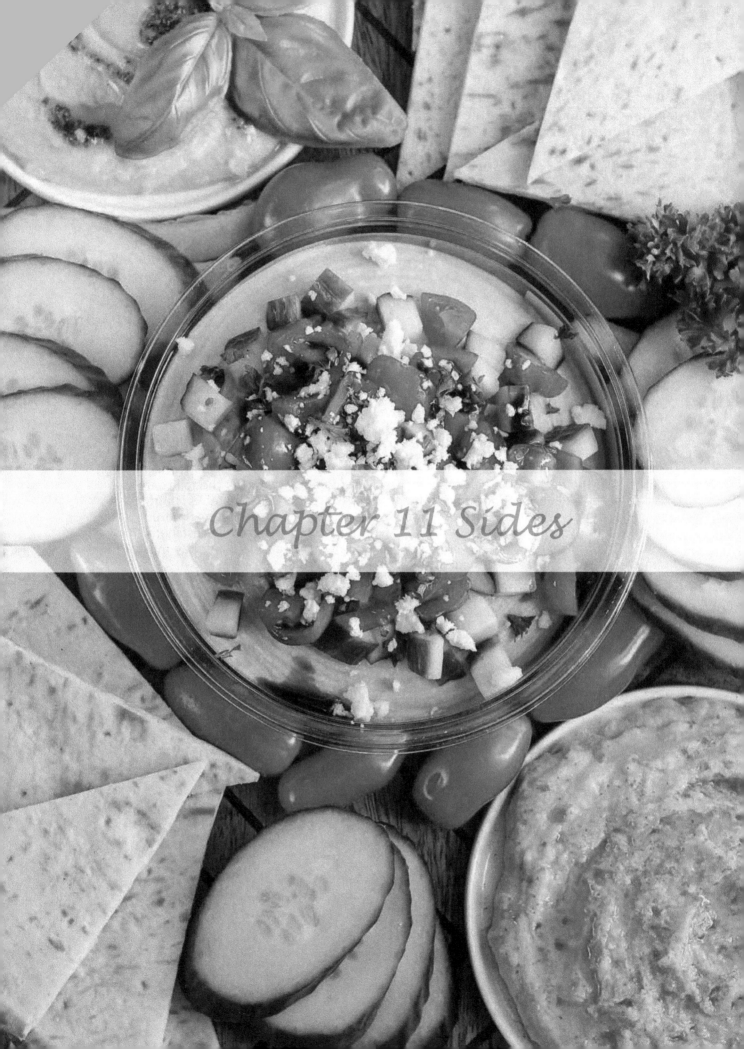

Chapter 11 Sides

Spicy Wilted Greens
Prep time: 10 minutes | Cook time: 5 minutes | Serves 2

1 tablespoon olive oil
2 garlic cloves, minced
3 cups sliced greens (kale, spinach, chard, beet greens, dandelion greens, or a combination)
Pinch salt
Pinch red pepper flakes (or more to taste)

1. Heat the olive oil in a sauté pan over medium-high heat. Add garlic and sauté for 30 seconds, or just until it's fragrant.
2. Add the greens, salt, and pepper flakes and stir to combine. Let the greens wilt, but do not overcook. Remove the pan from the heat and serve.

Per Serving
calories: 91 | fat: 7g | protein: 1g
carbs: 7g | fiber: 3g | sodium: 111mg

Mediterranean Bruschetta Hummus Platter
Prep time: 15 minutes | Cook time: 0 minutes | Serves 6

½ cup finely diced fresh tomato
⅓ cup finely diced seedless English cucumber
1 teaspoon extra-virgin olive oil
1 (10-ounce / 283-g) container plain hummus
2 tablespoons balsamic glaze
2 tablespoons crumbled feta cheese
1 tablespoon fresh chopped parsley or basil
¼ cup Herbed Olive Oil
4 warmed pitas, cut into wedges, for serving
Carrot sticks, for serving
Celery sticks, for serving
Sliced bell peppers, for serving
Broccoli, for serving
Purple cauliflower, for serving

1. In a small bowl, mix the tomato and cucumber and toss with the olive oil. Pile the cucumber mixture over a fresh container of hummus. Drizzle the hummus and vegetables with the balsamic glaze. Top with crumbled feta and fresh parsley.
2. Put the hummus on a large cutting board. Pour the Herbed Olive Oil in a small bowl and put it on the cutting board. Surround the bowls with the pita wedges and cut carrot sticks, celery sticks, sliced bell peppers, broccoli, and cauliflower.

Per Serving
calories: 345 | fat: 19g | protein: 9g
carbs: 32g | fiber: 3g | sodium: 473mg

Garlic Broccoli with Artichoke Hearts
Prep time: 5 minutes | Cook time: 10 minutes | Serves 4

2 pounds (907 g) fresh broccoli rabe
½ cup extra-virgin olive oil, divided
3 garlic cloves, finely minced
1 teaspoon salt
1 teaspoon red pepper flakes
1 (13¾-ounce / 390-g) can artichoke hearts, drained and quartered
1 tablespoon water
2 tablespoons red wine vinegar
Freshly ground black pepper, to taste

1. Trim away any thick lower stems and yellow leaves from the broccoli rabe and discard. Cut into individual florets with a couple inches of thin stem attached.
2. In a large skillet, heat ¼ cup olive oil over medium-high heat. Add the trimmed broccoli, garlic, salt, and red pepper flakes and sauté for 5 minutes, until the broccoli begins to soften. Add the artichoke hearts and sauté for another 2 minutes.
3. Add the water and reduce the heat to low. Cover and simmer until the broccoli stems are tender, 3 to 5 minutes.
4. In a small bowl, whisk together remaining ¼ cup olive oil and the vinegar. Drizzle over the broccoli and artichokes. Season with ground black pepper, if desired.

Per Serving
calories: 358 | fat: 35g | protein: 11g
carbs: 18g | fiber: 10g | sodium: 918mg

Lemon and Thyme Roasted Vegetables

Prep time: 20 minutes | Cook time: 50 minutes | Serves 2

1 head garlic, cloves split apart, unpeeled
2 tablespoons olive oil, divided
2 medium carrots
¼ pound (113 g) asparagus
6 Brussels sprouts
2 cups cauliflower florets
½ pint cherry or grape tomatoes
½ fresh lemon, sliced
Salt and freshly ground black pepper, to taste
3 sprigs fresh thyme or ½ teaspoon dried thyme
Freshly squeezed lemon juice

1. Preheat oven to 375ºF (190ºC) and set the rack to the middle position. Line a sheet pan with parchment paper or foil.
2. Place the garlic cloves in a small piece of foil and wrap lightly to enclose them, but don't seal the package. Drizzle with 1 teaspoon of olive oil. Place the foil packet on the sheet pan and roast for 30 minutes while you prepare the remaining vegetables.
3. While garlic is roasting, clean, peel, and trim vegetables: Cut carrots into strips, ½-inch wide and 3 to 4 inches long; snap tough ends off asparagus; trim tough ends off the Brussels sprouts and cut in half if they are large; trim cauliflower into 2-inch florets; keep tomatoes whole. The vegetables should be cut into pieces of similar size for even roasting.
4. Place all vegetables and the lemon slices into a large mixing bowl. Drizzle with the remaining 5 teaspoons of olive oil and season generously with salt and pepper.
5. Increase the oven temperature to 400ºF (205ºC).
6. Arrange the vegetables on the sheet pan in a single layer, leaving the packet of garlic cloves on the pan. Roast for 20 minutes, turning occasionally, until tender.
7. When the vegetables are tender, remove from the oven and sprinkle with thyme leaves. Let the garlic cloves sit until cool enough to handle, and then remove the skins. Leave them whole, or gently mash.
8. Toss garlic with the vegetables and an additional squeeze of fresh lemon juice.

Per Serving
calories: 256 | fat: 15g | protein: 7g
carbs: 31g | fiber: 9g | sodium: 168mg

Roasted Parmesan Rosemary Potatoes

Prep time: 10 minutes | Cook time: 55 minutes | Serves 2

12 ounces (340 g) red potatoes (3 to 4 small potatoes)
1 tablespoon olive oil
½ teaspoon garlic powder
¼ teaspoon salt
1 tablespoon grated Parmesan cheese
1 teaspoon minced fresh rosemary (from 1 sprig)

1. Preheat the oven to 425ºF (220ºC) and set the rack to the bottom position. Line a baking sheet with parchment paper. (Do not use foil, as the potatoes will stick.)
2. Scrub the potatoes and dry them well. Dice into 1-inch pieces.
3. In a mixing bowl, combine the potatoes, olive oil, garlic powder, and salt. Toss well to coat.
4. Lay the potatoes on the parchment paper and roast for 10 minutes. Flip the potatoes over and return to the oven for 10 more minutes.
5. Check the potatoes to make sure they are golden brown on the top and bottom. Toss them again, turn the heat down to 350ºF (180ºC), and roast for 30 minutes more.
6. When the potatoes are golden, crispy, and cooked through, sprinkle the Parmesan cheese over them and toss again. Return to the oven for 3 minutes to let the cheese melt a bit.
7. Remove from the oven and sprinkle with the fresh rosemary.

Per Serving
calories: 193 | fat: 8g | protein: 5g
carbs: 28g | fiber: 3g | sodium: 334mg

Romano Broccolini

Prep time: 5 minutes | Cook time: 10 minutes | Serves 2

1 bunch broccolini (about 5 ounces / 142 g)
1 tablespoon olive oil
½ teaspoon garlic powder
¼ teaspoon salt
2 tablespoons grated Romano cheese

1. Preheat the oven to 400ºF (205ºC) and set the oven rack to the middle position. Line a sheet pan with parchment paper or foil.
2. Slice the tough ends off the broccolini and place in a medium bowl. Add the olive oil, garlic powder, and salt and toss to combine. Arrange broccolini on the lined sheet pan.
3. Roast for 7 minutes, flipping pieces over halfway through the roasting time.
4. Remove the pan from the oven and sprinkle the cheese over the broccolini. With a pair of tongs, carefully flip the pieces over to coat all sides. Return to the oven for another 2 to 3 minutes, or until the cheese melts and starts to turn golden.

Per Serving
calories: 114 | fat: 9g | protein: 4g
carbs: 5g | fiber: 2g | sodium: 400mg

Balsamic Brussels Sprouts and Delicata Squash

Prep time: 10 minutes | Cook time: 30 minutes | Serves 2

½ pound (227 g) Brussels sprouts, ends trimmed and outer leaves removed
1 medium delicata squash, halved lengthwise, seeded, and cut into 1-inch pieces
1 cup fresh cranberries
2 teaspoons olive oil
Salt and freshly ground black pepper, to taste
½ cup balsamic vinegar
2 tablespoons roasted pumpkin seeds
2 tablespoons fresh pomegranate arils (seeds)

1. Preheat oven to 400ºF (205ºC) and set the rack to the middle position. Line a sheet pan with parchment paper.
2. Combine the Brussels sprouts, squash, and cranberries in a large bowl. Drizzle with olive oil, and season liberally with salt and pepper. Toss well to coat and arrange in a single layer on the sheet pan.
3. Roast for 30 minutes, turning vegetables halfway through, or until Brussels sprouts turn brown and crisp in spots and squash has golden-brown spots.
4. While vegetables are roasting, prepare the balsamic glaze by simmering the vinegar for 10 to 12 minutes, or until mixture has reduced to about ¼ cup and turns a syrupy consistency.
5. Remove the vegetables from the oven, drizzle with balsamic syrup, and sprinkle with pumpkin seeds and pomegranate arils before serving.

Per Serving
calories: 201 | fat: 7g | protein: 6g
carbs: 21g | fiber: 8g | sodium: 34mg

Honey Roasted Rainbow Carrots

Prep time: 10 minutes | Cook time: 20 minutes | Serves 2

½ pound (227 g) rainbow carrots (about 4)
2 tablespoons fresh orange juice
1 tablespoon honey
½ teaspoon coriander
Pinch salt

1. Preheat oven to 400ºF (205ºC) and set the oven rack to the middle position.
2. Peel the carrots and cut them lengthwise into slices of even thickness. Place them in a large bowl.
3. In a small bowl, mix together the orange juice, honey, coriander, and salt.
4. Pour the orange juice mixture over the carrots and toss well to coat.
5. Spread carrots onto a baking dish in a single layer.
6. Roast for 15 to 20 minutes, or until fork-tender.

Per Serving
calories: 85 | fat: 0g | protein: 1g
carbs: 21g | fiber: 3g | sodium: 156mg

Garlicky Roasted Grape Tomatoes

Prep time: 10 minutes | Cook time: 45 minutes | Serves 2

1 pint grape tomatoes
10 whole garlic cloves, skins removed
¼ cup olive oil
½ teaspoon salt
1 fresh rosemary sprig
1 fresh thyme sprig

1. Preheat oven to 350ºF (180ºC).
2. Toss tomatoes, garlic cloves, oil, salt, and herb sprigs in a baking dish.
3. Roast tomatoes until they are soft and begin to caramelize, about 45 minutes.
4. Remove herbs before serving.

Per Serving

calories: 271 | fat: 26g | protein: 3g
carbs: 12g | fiber: 3g | sodium: 593mg

Roasted Lemon Tahini Cauliflower

Prep time: 10 minutes | Cook time: 20 minutes | Serves 2

½ large head cauliflower, stemmed and broken into florets (about 3 cups)
1 tablespoon olive oil
2 tablespoons tahini
2 tablespoons freshly squeezed lemon juice
1 teaspoon harissa paste
Pinch salt

1. Preheat the oven to 400ºF (205ºC) and set the rack to the lowest position. Line a sheet pan with parchment paper or foil.
2. Toss the cauliflower florets with the olive oil in a large bowl and transfer to the sheet pan. Reserve the bowl to make the tahini sauce.
3. Roast the cauliflower for 15 minutes, turning it once or twice, until it starts to turn golden.
4. In the same bowl, combine the tahini, lemon juice, harissa, and salt.
5. When the cauliflower is tender, remove it from the oven and toss it with the tahini sauce. Return to the sheet pan and roast for 5 minutes more.

Per Serving

calories: 205 | fat: 15g | protein: 7g
carbs: 15g | fiber: 7g | sodium: 161mg

Pistachio Citrus Asparagus

Prep time: 10 minutes | Cook time: 15 minutes | Serves 4

5 tablespoons extra-virgin olive oil, divided
Zest and juice of 2 clementines or 1 orange (about ¼ cup juice and 1 tablespoon zest)
Zest and juice of 1 lemon
1 tablespoon red
wine vinegar
1 teaspoon salt, divided
¼ teaspoon freshly ground black pepper
½ cup shelled pistachios
1 pound (454 g) fresh asparagus
1 tablespoon water

1. In a small bowl, whisk together 4 tablespoons olive oil, the clementine and lemon juices and zests, vinegar, ½ teaspoon salt, and pepper. Set aside.
2. In a medium dry skillet, toast the pistachios over medium-high heat until lightly browned, 2 to 3 minutes, being careful not to let them burn. Transfer to a cutting board and coarsely chop. Set aside.
3. Trim the rough ends off the asparagus, usually the last 1 to 2 inches of each spear. In a skillet, heat the remaining 1 tablespoon olive oil over medium-high heat. Add the asparagus and sauté for 2 to 3 minutes. Sprinkle with the remaining ½ teaspoon salt and add the water. Reduce the heat to medium-low, cover, and cook until tender, another 2 to 4 minutes, depending on the thickness of the spears.
4. Transfer the cooked asparagus to a serving dish. Add the pistachios to the dressing and whisk to combine. Pour the dressing over the warm asparagus and toss to coat.

Per Serving

calories: 284 | fat: 24g | protein: 6g
carbs: 11g | fiber: 4g | sodium: 594mg

Sautéed Riced Cauliflower

Prep time: 5 minutes | Cook time: 5 minutes | Serves 6 to 8

1 small head cauliflower, broken into florets
¼ cup extra-virgin olive oil
2 garlic cloves, finely minced

1½ teaspoons salt
½ teaspoon freshly ground black pepper

1. Place the florets in a food processor and pulse several times, until the cauliflower is the consistency of rice or couscous.
2. In a large skillet, heat the olive oil over medium-high heat. Add the cauliflower, garlic, salt, and pepper and sauté for 5 minutes, just to take the crunch out but not enough to let the cauliflower become soggy.
3. Remove the cauliflower from the skillet and place in a bowl until ready to use. Toss with chopped herbs and additional olive oil for a simple side, top with sautéed veggies and protein, or use in your favorite recipe.

Per Serving
calories: 92 | fat: 8g | protein: 1g | carbs: 3g | fiber: 0g | sodium: 595mg

Herb-Roasted Vegetables

Prep time: 15 minutes | Cook time: 45 minutes | Serves 6

Nonstick cooking spray
2 eggplants, peeled and sliced ⅛ inch thick
1 zucchini, sliced ¼ inch thick
1 yellow summer squash, sliced ¼ inch thick
2 Roma tomatoes, sliced ⅛ inch thick
¼ cup, plus 2 tablespoons extra-virgin olive

oil, divided
1 tablespoon garlic powder
¼ teaspoon dried oregano
¼ teaspoon dried basil
¼ teaspoon salt
Freshly ground black pepper, to taste

1. Preheat the oven to 400ºF (205ºC).
2. Spray a 9-by-13-inch baking dish with cooking spray. In the dish, toss the eggplant, zucchini, squash, and tomatoes with 2 tablespoons oil, garlic powder, oregano, basil, salt, and pepper.
3. Standing the vegetables up (like little soldiers), alternate layers of eggplant, zucchini, squash, and Roma tomato.
4. Drizzle the top with the remaining ¼ cup of olive oil.
5. Bake, uncovered, for 40 to 45 minutes, or until vegetables are golden brown.

Per Serving
calories: 186 | fat: 14g | protein: 3g | carbs: 15g | fiber: 5g | sodium: 110mg

Spinach and Zucchini Lasagna

Prep time: 15 minutes | Cook time: 1 hour | Serves 8

½ cup extra-virgin olive oil, divided
4 to 5 medium zucchini squash
1 teaspoon salt
8 ounces (227 g) frozen spinach, thawed and well drained (about 1 cup)
2 cups whole-milk ricotta cheese
¼ cup chopped fresh basil or 2 teaspoons dried basil

1 teaspoon garlic powder
½ teaspoon freshly ground black pepper
2 cups shredded fresh whole-milk Mozzarella cheese
1¾ cups shredded Parmesan cheese
½ (24-ounce / 680-g) jar low-sugar marinara sauce (less than 5 grams sugar)

1. Preheat the oven to 425ºF (220ºC).
2. Line two baking sheets with parchment paper or aluminum foil and drizzle each with 2 tablespoons olive oil, spreading evenly.
3. Slice the zucchini lengthwise into ¼-inch-thick long slices and place on the prepared baking sheet in a single layer. Sprinkle with ½ teaspoon salt per sheet. Bake until softened, but not mushy, 15 to 18 minutes. Remove from the oven and allow to cool slightly before assembling the lasagna.
4. Reduce the oven temperature to 375ºF (190ºC).
5. While the zucchini cooks, prep the filling. In a large bowl, combine the spinach, ricotta, basil, garlic powder, and pepper. In a small bowl, mix together the Mozzarella and Parmesan cheeses. In a medium bowl, combine the marinara sauce and remaining ¼ cup olive oil and stir to fully incorporate the oil into sauce.
6. To assemble the lasagna, spoon a third of the marinara sauce mixture into the bottom of a 9-by-13-inch glass baking dish and spread evenly. Place 1 layer of softened zucchini slices to fully cover the sauce, then add a third of the ricotta-spinach mixture and spread evenly on top of the zucchini. Sprinkle a third of the Mozzarella-Parmesan mixture on top of the ricotta. Repeat with 2 more cycles of these layers: marinara, zucchini, ricotta-spinach, then cheese blend.
7. Bake until the cheese is bubbly and melted, 30 to 35 minutes. Turn the broiler to low and broil until the top is golden brown, about 5 minutes. Remove from the oven and allow to cool slightly before slicing.

Per Serving
calories: 521 | fat: 41g | protein: 25g | carbs: 13g | fiber: 3g | sodium: 712mg

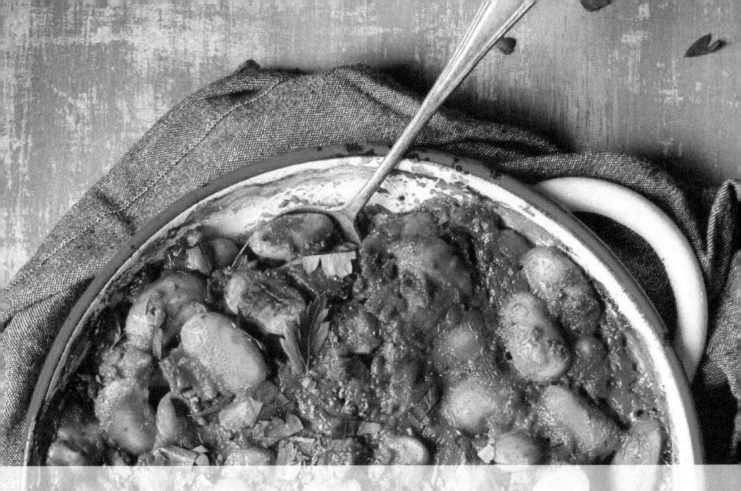
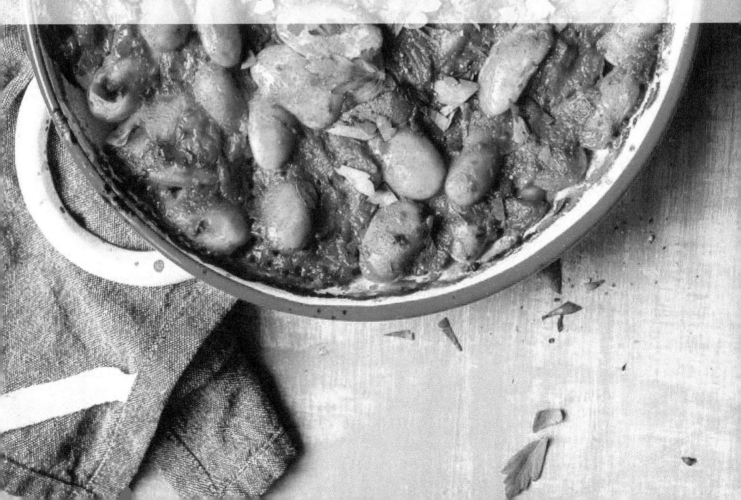

Chapter 12 Beans

Baked Sweet Potato Black Bean Burgers

Prep time: 10 minutes | Cook time: 10 minutes | Serves 4

1 (15-ounce / 425-g) can black beans, drained and rinsed
1 cup mashed sweet potato
½ teaspoon dried oregano
¼ teaspoon dried thyme
¼ teaspoon dried marjoram

1 garlic clove, minced
¼ teaspoon salt
¼ teaspoon black pepper
1 tablespoon lemon juice
1 cup cooked brown rice
¼ to ½ cup whole wheat bread crumbs
1 tablespoon olive oil

For Serving:

Whole wheat buns or whole wheat pitas
Plain Greek yogurt
Avocado

Lettuce
Tomato
Red onion

1. Preheat the air fryer to 380ºF (193ºC).
2. In a large bowl, use the back of a fork to mash the black beans until there are no large pieces left.
3. Add the mashed sweet potato, oregano, thyme, marjoram, garlic, salt, pepper, and lemon juice, and mix until well combined.
4. Stir in the cooked rice.
5. Add in ¼ cup of the whole wheat bread crumbs and stir. Check to see if the mixture is dry enough to form patties. If it seems too wet and loose, add an additional ¼ cup bread crumbs and stir.
6. Form the dough into 4 patties. Place them into the air fryer basket in a single layer, making sure that they don't touch each other.
7. Brush half of the olive oil onto the patties and bake for 5 minutes.
8. Flip the patties over, brush the other side with the remaining oil, and bake for an additional 4 to 5 minutes.
9. Serve on toasted whole wheat buns or whole wheat pitas with a spoonful of yogurt and avocado, lettuce, tomato, and red onion as desired.

Per Serving
calories: 263 | fat: 5g | protein: 9g
carbs: 47g | fiber: 8g | sodium: 247mg

Oregano Lentil and Carrot Patties

Prep time: 15 minutes | Cook time: 10 minutes | Serves 4

1 cup cooked brown lentils
¼ cup fresh parsley leaves
½ cup shredded carrots
¼ red onion, minced
¼ red bell pepper, minced
1 jalapeño, seeded and minced
2 garlic cloves, minced
1 egg
2 tablespoons lemon

juice
2 tablespoons olive oil, divided
½ teaspoon onion powder
½ teaspoon smoked paprika
½ teaspoon dried oregano
¼ teaspoon salt
¼ teaspoon black pepper
½ cup whole wheat bread crumbs

For Serving:

Whole wheat buns or whole wheat pitas
Plain Greek yogurt

Tomato
Lettuce
Red Onion

1. Preheat the air fryer to 380ºF (193ºC).
2. In a food processor, pulse the lentils and parsley mostly smooth. (You will want some bits of lentils in the mixture.)
3. Pour the lentils into a large bowl, and combine with the carrots, onion, bell pepper, jalapeño, garlic, egg, lemon juice, and 1 tablespoon olive oil.
4. Add the onion powder, paprika, oregano, salt, pepper, and bread crumbs. Stir everything together until the seasonings and bread crumbs are well distributed.
5. Form the dough into 4 patties. Place them into the air fryer basket in a single layer, making sure that they don't touch each other. Brush the remaining 1 tablespoon of olive oil over the patties.
6. Bake for 5 minutes. Flip the patties over and bake for an additional 5 minutes.
7. Serve on toasted whole wheat buns or whole wheat pitas with a spoonful of yogurt and lettuce, tomato, and red onion as desired.

Per Serving
calories: 206 | fat: 9g | protein: 8g
carbs: 25g | fiber: 6g | sodium: 384mg

Herb Lentil-Rice Balls
Prep time: 5 minutes | Cook time: 11 minutes | Serves 6

½ cup cooked green lentils
2 garlic cloves, minced
¼ white onion, minced
¼ cup parsley leaves
5 basil leaves
1 cup cooked brown rice
1 tablespoon lemon juice
1 tablespoon olive oil
½ teaspoon salt

1. Preheat the air fryer to 380ºF (193ºC).
2. In a food processor, pulse the cooked lentils with the garlic, onion, parsley, and basil until mostly smooth. (You will want some bits of lentils in the mixture.)
3. Pour the lentil mixture into a large bowl, and stir in brown rice, lemon juice, olive oil, and salt. Stir until well combined.
4. Form the rice mixture into 1-inch balls. Place the rice balls in a single layer in the air fryer basket, making sure that they don't touch each other.
5. Fry for 6 minutes. Turn the rice balls and then fry for an additional 4 to 5 minutes, or until browned on all sides.

Per Serving
calories: 80 | fat: 3g | protein: 2g
carbs: 12g | fiber: 2g | sodium: 198mg

Greek Baked Two Beans
Prep time: 15 minutes | Cook time: 30 minutes | Serves 4

Olive oil cooking spray
1 (15-ounce / 425-g) can cannellini beans, drained and rinsed
1 (15-ounce / 425-g) can great northern beans, drained and rinsed
½ yellow onion, diced
1 (8-ounce) can tomato sauce
1½ tablespoons raw honey
¼ cup olive oil
2 garlic cloves, minced
2 tablespoons chopped fresh dill
½ teaspoon salt
½ teaspoon black pepper
1 bay leaf
1 tablespoon balsamic vinegar
2 ounces (57 g) feta cheese, crumbled, for serving

1. Preheat the air fryer to 360ºF (182ºC). Lightly coat the inside of a 5-cup capacity casserole dish with olive oil cooking spray. (The shape of the casserole dish will depend upon the size of the air fryer, but it needs to be able to hold at least 5 cups.)
2. In a large bowl, combine all ingredients except the feta cheese and stir until well combined.
3. Pour the bean mixture into the prepared casserole dish.
4. Bake in the air fryer for 30 minutes.
5. Remove from the air fryer and remove and discard the bay leaf. Sprinkle crumbled feta over the top before serving.

Per Serving
calories: 397 | fat: 18g | protein: 14g
carbs: 48g | fiber: 16g | sodium: 886mg

Black-Eyed Peas Salad with Walnuts
Prep time: 10 minutes | Cook time: 0 minutes | Serves 4 to 6

3 tablespoons extra-virgin olive oil
3 tablespoons dukkah, divided
2 tablespoons lemon juice
2 tablespoons pomegranate molasses
¼ teaspoon salt, or more to taste
⅛ teaspoon pepper,
or more to taste
2 (15-ounce / 425-g) cans black-eyed peas, rinsed
½ cup pomegranate seeds
½ cup minced fresh parsley
½ cup walnuts, toasted and chopped
4 scallions, sliced thinly

1. In a large bowl, whisk together the olive oil, 2 tablespoons of the dukkah, lemon juice, pomegranate molasses, salt and pepper.
2. Stir in the remaining ingredients. Season with salt and pepper.
3. Sprinkle with the remaining 1 tablespoon of the dukkah before serving.

Per Serving
calories: 155 | fat: 11g | protein: 2g
carbs: 12g | fiber: 2g | sodium: 105mg

White Cannellini Bean Stew

Prep time: 10 minutes | Cook time: 30 minutes | Serves 4 to 6

3 tablespoons extra-virgin olive oil
1 large onion, chopped
1 (15-ounce / 425-g) can diced tomatoes
2 (15-ounce / 425-g) cans white cannellini beans

1 cup carrots, chopped
4 cups vegetable broth
1 teaspoon salt
1 (1-pound / 454-g) bag baby spinach, washed

1. In a large pot over medium heat, cook the olive oil and onion for 5 minutes.
2. Add the tomatoes, beans, carrots, broth, and salt. Stir and cook for 20 minutes.
3. Add the spinach, a handful at a time, and cook for 5 minutes, until the spinach has wilted.
4. Serve warm.

Per Serving
calories: 356 | fat: 12g | protein: 15g
carbs: 47g | fiber: 16g | sodium: 1832mg

Turkish-Inspired Pinto Bean Salad

Prep time: 10 minutes | Cook time: 3 minutes | Serves 4 to 6

¼ cup extra-virgin olive oil, divided
3 garlic cloves, lightly crushed and peeled
2 (15-ounce / 425-g) cans pinto beans, rinsed
2 cups plus 1 tablespoon water
Salt and pepper, to taste
¼ cup tahini
3 tablespoons lemon juice

1 tablespoon ground dried Aleppo pepper, plus extra for serving
8 ounces (227 g) cherry tomatoes, halved
¼ red onion, sliced thinly
½ cup fresh parsley leaves
2 hard-cooked large eggs, quartered
1 tablespoon toasted sesame seeds

1. Add 1 tablespoon of the olive oil and garlic to a medium saucepan over medium heat. Cook for about 3 minutes, stirring constantly, or until the garlic turns golden but not brown.

2. Add the beans, 2 cups of the water and 1 teaspoon salt and bring to a simmer. Remove from the heat, cover and let sit for 20 minutes. Drain the beans and discard the garlic.
3. In a large bowl, whisk together the remaining 3 tablespoons of the oil, tahini, lemon juice, Aleppo, the remaining 1 tablespoon of the water and ¼ teaspoon salt. Stir in the beans, tomatoes, onion and parsley. Season with salt and pepper to taste.
4. Transfer to a serving platter and top with the eggs. Sprinkle with the sesame seeds and extra Aleppo before serving.

Per Serving
calories: 402 | fat: 18g | protein: 16g
carbs: 44g | fiber: 11g | sodium: 456mg

White Bean Lettuce Wraps

Prep time: 10 minutes | Cook time: 9 minutes | Serves 4

1 tablespoon extra-virgin olive oil
½ cup diced red onion
¾ cup chopped fresh tomatoes
¼ teaspoon freshly ground black pepper
1 (15-ounce / 425-g) can cannellini or

great northern beans, drained and rinsed
¼ cup finely chopped fresh curly parsley
½ cup lemony garlic hummus or ½ cup prepared hummus
8 romaine lettuce leaves

1. In a large skillet over medium heat, heat the oil. Add the onion and cook for 3 minutes, stirring occasionally. Add the tomatoes and pepper and cook for 3 more minutes, stirring occasionally. Add the beans and cook for 3 more minutes, stirring occasionally. Remove from the heat, and mix in the parsley.
2. Spread 1 tablespoon of hummus over each lettuce leaf. Evenly spread the warm bean mixture down the center of each leaf. Fold one side of the lettuce leaf over the filling lengthwise, then fold over the other side to make a wrap and serve.

Per Serving
calories: 188 | fat: 5g | protein: 10g
carbs: 28g | fiber: 9g | sodium: 115mg

Bean Balls with Marinara

Prep time: 15 minutes | Cook time: 30 minutes | Serves 2 to 4

Bean Balls:

1 tablespoon extra-virgin olive oil
½ yellow onion, minced
1 teaspoon fennel seeds
2 teaspoons dried oregano
½ teaspoon crushed red pepper flakes

1 teaspoon garlic powder
1 (15-ounce / 425-g) can white beans (cannellini or navy), drained and rinsed
½ cup whole-grain bread crumbs
Sea salt and ground black pepper, to taste

Marinara:

1 tablespoon extra-virgin olive oil
3 garlic cloves, minced
Handful basil leaves

1 (28-ounce / 794-g) can chopped tomatoes with juice reserved
Sea salt, to taste

Make the Bean Balls

1. Preheat the oven to 350°F (180°C). Line a baking sheet with parchment paper.
2. Heat the olive oil in a nonstick skillet over medium heat until shimmering.
3. Add the onion and sauté for 5 minutes or until translucent.
4. Sprinkle with fennel seeds, oregano, red pepper flakes, and garlic powder, then cook for 1 minute or until aromatic.
5. Pour the sautéed mixture in a food processor and add the beans and bread crumbs. Sprinkle with salt and ground black pepper, then pulse to combine well and the mixture holds together.
6. Shape the mixture into balls with a 2-ounce (57-g) cookie scoop, then arrange the balls on the baking sheet.
7. Bake in the preheated oven for 30 minutes or until lightly browned. Flip the balls halfway through the cooking time.

Make the Marinara

1. While baking the bean balls, heat the olive oil in a saucepan over medium-high heat until shimmering.
2. Add the garlic and basil and sauté for 2 minutes or until fragrant.
3. Fold in the tomatoes and juice. Bring to a boil. Reduce the heat to low. Put the lid on and simmer for 15 minutes. Sprinkle with salt.

4. Transfer the bean balls on a large plate and baste with marinara before serving.

Per Serving

calories: 351 | fat: 16g | protein: 11g
carbs: 42g | fiber: 10g | sodium: 377mg

Turmeric-Spiced Organic Chickpeas

Prep time: 10 minutes | Cook time: 30 minutes | Serves 4

2 (15-ounce / 425-g) cans organic chickpeas, drained and rinsed
3 tablespoons extra-virgin olive oil
2 teaspoons Turkish or smoked paprika
2 teaspoons turmeric

½ teaspoon dried oregano
½ teaspoon salt
¼ teaspoon ground ginger
⅛ teaspoon ground white pepper (optional)

1. Preheat the oven to 400°F (205°C). Line a baking sheet with parchment paper and set aside.
2. Completely dry the chickpeas. Lay the chickpeas out on a baking sheet, roll them around with paper towels, and allow them to air-dry. I usually let them dry for at least 2½ hours, but can also be left to dry overnight.
3. In a medium bowl, combine the olive oil, paprika, turmeric, oregano, salt, ginger, and white pepper (if using).
4. Add the dry chickpeas to the bowl and toss to combine.
5. Put the chickpeas on the prepared baking sheet and cook for 30 minutes, or until the chickpeas turn golden brown. At 15 minutes, move the chickpeas around on the baking sheet to avoid burning. Check every 10 minutes in case the chickpeas begin to crisp up before the full cooking time has elapsed.
6. Remove from the oven and set them aside to cool.

Per Serving (½ cup)

calories: 308 | fat: 12g | protein: 11g
carbs: 40g | fiber: 10g | sodium: 292mg

Chili Black Bean with Mangoes

Prep time: 10 minutes | Cook time: 10 minutes | Serves 4

2 tablespoons coconut oil
1 onion, chopped
2 (15-ounce / 425-g) cans black beans, drained and rinsed
1 tablespoon chili powder
1 teaspoon sea salt
¼ teaspoon freshly ground black pepper
1 cup water
2 ripe mangoes, sliced thinly
¼ cup chopped fresh cilantro, divided
¼ cup sliced scallions, divided

1. Heat the coconut oil in a pot over high heat until melted.
2. Put the onion in the pot and sauté for 5 minutes or until translucent.
3. Add the black beans to the pot. Sprinkle with chili powder, salt, and ground black pepper. Pour in the water. Stir to mix well.
4. Bring to a boil. Reduce the heat to low, then simmering for 5 minutes or until the beans are tender.
5. Turn off the heat and mix in the mangoes, then garnish with scallions and cilantro before serving.

Per Serving
calories: 277 | fat: 9g | protein: 4g
carbs: 45g | fiber: 7g | sodium: 647mg

Garbanzo and Fava Bean Fūl

Prep time: 10 minutes | Cook time: 10 minutes | Serves 6

1 (16-ounce / 454-g) can garbanzo beans, rinsed and drained
1 (15-ounce / 425-g) can fava beans, rinsed and drained
3 cups water
½ cup lemon juice
3 cloves garlic, peeled and minced
1 teaspoon salt
3 tablespoons extra-virgin olive oil

1. In a 3-quart pot over medium heat, cook the garbanzo beans, fava beans, and water for 10 minutes.
2. Reserving 1 cup of the liquid from the cooked beans, drain the beans and put them in a bowl.
3. Mix the reserved liquid, lemon juice, minced garlic, and salt together and add to the beans in the bowl. Using a potato masher, mash up about half the beans in the bowl.
4. After mashing half the beans, give the mixture one more stir to make sure the beans are evenly mixed.
5. Drizzle the olive oil over the top.
6. Serve warm or cold with pita bread.

Per Serving
calories: 199 | fat: 9g | protein: 10g
carbs: 25g | fiber: 9g | sodium: 395mg

Mashed Beans with Cumin

Prep time: 10 minutes | Cook time: 10 to 12 minutes | Serves 4 to 6

1 tablespoon extra-virgin olive oil, plus extra for serving
4 garlic cloves, minced
1 teaspoon ground cumin
2 (15-ounce / 425-g) cans fava beans
3 tablespoons tahini
2 tablespoons lemon juice, plus lemon
wedges for serving
Salt and pepper, to taste
1 tomato, cored and cut into ½-inch pieces
1 small onion, chopped finely
2 hard-cooked large eggs, chopped
2 tablespoons minced fresh parsley

1. Add the olive oil, garlic and cumin to a medium saucepan over medium heat. Cook for about 2 minutes, or until fragrant.
2. Stir in the beans with their liquid and tahini. Bring to a simmer and cook for 8 to 10 minutes, or until the liquid thickens slightly.
3. Turn off the heat, mash the beans to a coarse consistency with a potato masher. Stir in the lemon juice and 1 teaspoon pepper. Season with salt and pepper.
4. Transfer the mashed beans to a serving dish. Top with the tomato, onion, eggs and parsley. Drizzle with the extra olive oil.
5. Serve with the lemon wedges.

Per Serving
calories: 125 | fat: 8g | protein: 5g
carbs: 9g | fiber: 3g | sodium: 131mg

Lentil Stuffed Tomatoes
Prep time: 10 minutes | Cook time: 15 minutes | Serves 4

4 tomatoes
½ cup cooked red lentils
1 garlic clove, minced
1 tablespoon minced red onion
4 basil leaves, minced

¼ teaspoon salt
¼ teaspoon black pepper
4 ounces (113 g) goat cheese
2 tablespoons shredded Parmesan cheese

1. Preheat the air fryer to 380ºF (193ºC).
2. Slice the top off of each tomato.
3. Using a knife and spoon, cut and scoop out half of the flesh inside of the tomato. Place it into a medium bowl.
4. To the bowl with the tomato, add the cooked lentils, garlic, onion, basil, salt, pepper, and goat cheese. Stir until well combined.
5. Spoon the filling into the scooped-out cavity of each of the tomatoes, then top each one with ½ tablespoon of shredded Parmesan cheese.
6. Place the tomatoes in a single layer in the air fryer basket and bake for 15 minutes.

Per Serving
calories: 138 | fat: 7g | protein: 9g
carbs: 11g | fiber: 4g | sodium: 317mg

Italian-Style Baked Beans
Prep time: 10 minutes | Cook time: 15 minutes | Serves 6

2 teaspoons extra-virgin olive oil
½ cup minced onion
1 (12-ounce / 340-g) can low-sodium tomato paste
¼ cup red wine vinegar

2 tablespoons honey
¼ teaspoon ground cinnamon
½ cup water
2 (15-ounce / 425-g) cans cannellini or great northern beans, undrained

1. In a medium saucepan over medium heat, heat the oil. Add the onion and cook for 5 minutes, stirring frequently. Add the tomato paste, vinegar, honey, cinnamon, and water, and mix well. Turn the heat to low.

2. Drain and rinse one can of the beans in a colander and add to the saucepan. Pour the entire second can of beans (including the liquid) into the saucepan. Let it cook for 10 minutes, stirring occasionally, and serve.

Per Serving
calories: 290 | fat: 2g | protein: 15g
carbs: 53g | fiber: 11g | sodium: 647mg

Garlic and Parsley Chickpeas
Prep time: 10 minutes | Cook time: 18 to 20 minutes | Serves 4 to 6

¼ cup extra-virgin olive oil, divided
4 garlic cloves, sliced thinly
⅛ teaspoon red pepper flakes
1 onion, chopped finely
¼ teaspoon salt, plus more to taste

Black pepper, to taste
2 (15-ounce / 425-g) cans chickpeas, rinsed
1 cup vegetable broth
2 tablespoons minced fresh parsley
2 teaspoons lemon juice

1. Add 3 tablespoons of the olive oil, garlic, and pepper flakes to a skillet over medium heat. Cook for about 3 minutes, stirring constantly, or until the garlic turns golden but not brown.
2. Stir in the onion and ¼ teaspoon salt and cook for 5 to 7 minutes, or until softened and lightly browned.
3. Add the chickpeas and broth to the skillet and bring to a simmer. Reduce the heat to medium-low, cover, and cook for about 7 minutes, or until the chickpeas are cooked through and flavors meld.
4. Uncover, increase the heat to high and continue to cook for about 3 minutes more, or until nearly all liquid has evaporated.
5. Turn off the heat, stir in the parsley and lemon juice. Season to taste with salt and pepper and drizzle with remaining 1 tablespoon of the olive oil.
6. Serve warm.

Per Serving
calories: 220 | fat: 11g | protein: 6g
carbs: 24g | fiber: 6g | sodium: 467mg

Mediterranean Green Peas with Parmesan

Prep time: 15 minutes | Cook time: 25 minutes | Serves 8

1 cup cauliflower florets, fresh or frozen
½ white onion, roughly chopped
2 tablespoons olive oil
½ cup unsweetened almond milk
3 cups green peas, fresh or frozen
3 garlic cloves, minced
2 tablespoons fresh thyme leaves, chopped
1 teaspoon fresh rosemary leaves, chopped
½ teaspoon salt
½ teaspoon black pepper
Shredded Parmesan cheese, for garnish
Fresh parsley, for garnish

1. Preheat the air fryer to 380ºF (193ºC).
2. In a large bowl, combine the cauliflower florets and onion with the olive oil and toss well to coat.
3. Put the cauliflower-and-onion mixture into the air fryer basket in an even layer and bake for 15 minutes.
4. Transfer the cauliflower and onion to a food processor. Add the almond milk and pulse until smooth.
5. In a medium saucepan, combine the cauliflower purée, peas, garlic, thyme, rosemary, salt, and pepper and mix well. Cook over medium heat for an additional 10 minutes, stirring regularly.
6. Serve with a sprinkle of Parmesan cheese and chopped fresh parsley.

Per Serving
calories: 87 | fat: 4g | protein: 4g
carbs: 10g | fiber: 3g | sodium: 163mg

Garbanzo and Pita Casserole

Prep time: 10 minutes | Cook time: 10 minutes | Serves 4

4 cups Greek yogurt
3 cloves garlic, minced
1 teaspoon salt
2 (16-ounce / 454-g) cans garbanzo beans,
rinsed and drained
2 cups water
4 cups pita chips
5 tablespoons unsalted butter (optional)

1. In a large bowl, whisk together the yogurt, garlic, and salt. Set aside.
2. Put the garbanzo beans and water in a medium pot. Bring to a boil; let beans boil for about 5 minutes.
3. Pour the garbanzo beans and the liquid into a large casserole dish.
4. Top the beans with pita chips. Pour the yogurt sauce over the pita chip layer.
5. In a small saucepan, melt and brown the butter (if desired), about 3 minutes. Pour the brown butter over the yogurt sauce.

Per Serving
calories: 772 | fat: 36g | protein: 39g
carbs: 73g | fiber: 13g | sodium: 1003mg

Lentil Sloppy Joes

Prep time: 15 minutes | Cook time: 15 minutes | Serves 4

1 tablespoon extra-virgin olive oil
1 cup chopped onion
1 cup chopped bell pepper, any color
2 garlic cloves, minced
1 (15-ounce / 425-g) can lentils, drained and rinsed
1 (14½-ounce / 411-g) can low-sodium or no-salt-added diced
tomatoes, undrained
1 teaspoon ground cumin
1 teaspoon dried thyme
¼ teaspoon kosher or sea salt
4 whole-wheat pita breads, split open
1½ cups chopped seedless cucumber
1 cup chopped romaine lettuce

1. In a medium saucepan over medium-high heat, heat the oil. Add the onion and bell pepper and cook for 4 minutes, stirring frequently. Add the garlic and cook for 1 minute, stirring frequently. Add the lentils, tomatoes (with their liquid), cumin, thyme, and salt. Turn the heat to medium and cook, stirring occasionally, for 10 minutes, or until most of the liquid has evaporated.
2. Stuff the lentil mixture inside each pita. Lay the cucumbers and lettuce on top of the lentil mixture and serve.

Per Serving
calories: 241 | fat: 3g | protein: 13g
carbs: 43g | fiber: 12g | sodium: 317mg

French Green Lentils with Chard

Prep time: 15 minutes | Cook time: 20 minutes | Serves 6

2 tablespoons extra-virgin olive oil, plus extra for drizzling
12 ounces (340 g) Swiss chard, stems chopped fine, leaves sliced into ½-inch-wide strips
1 onion, chopped fine
½ teaspoon table salt
2 garlic cloves, minced
1 teaspoon minced fresh thyme or ¼ teaspoon dried

2½ cups water
1 cup French green lentils, picked over and rinsed
3 tablespoons whole-grain mustard
½ teaspoon grated lemon zest plus 1 teaspoon juice
3 tablespoons sliced almonds, toasted
2 tablespoons chopped fresh parsley

1. Using highest sauté function, heat oil in Instant Pot until shimmering. Add chard stems, onion, and salt and cook until vegetables are softened, about 5 minutes. Stir in garlic and thyme and cook until fragrant, about 30 seconds. Stir in water and lentils.
2. Lock lid in place and close pressure release valve. Select high pressure cook function and cook for 11 minutes. Turn off Instant Pot and let pressure release naturally for 15 minutes. Quick-release any remaining pressure, then carefully remove lid, allowing steam to escape away from you.
3. Stir chard leaves into lentils, 1 handful at a time, and let cook in residual heat until wilted, about 5 minutes. Stir in mustard and lemon zest and juice. Season with salt and pepper to taste. Transfer to serving dish, drizzle with extra oil, and sprinkle with almonds and parsley. Serve.

Per Serving
calories: 190 | fat: 8g | protein: 9g
carbs: 23g | fiber: 6g | sodium: 470mg

Chickpeas with Coriander and Sage

Prep time: 15 minutes | Cook time: 21 minutes | Serves 6 to 8

1½ tablespoons table salt, for brining
1 pound (454 g) dried chickpeas, picked over and rinsed
2 tablespoons extra-virgin olive oil, plus extra for drizzling
2 onions, halved and sliced thin
¼ teaspoon table salt
1 tablespoon coriander seeds, cracked

¼ to ½ teaspoon red pepper flakes
2½ cups chicken broth
¼ cup fresh sage leaves
2 bay leaves
1½ teaspoons grated lemon zest plus 2 teaspoons juice
2 tablespoons minced fresh parsley

1. Dissolve 1½ tablespoons salt in 2 quarts cold water in large container. Add chickpeas and soak at room temperature for at least 8 hours or up to 24 hours. Drain and rinse well.
2. Using highest sauté function, heat oil in Instant Pot until shimmering. Add onions and ¼ teaspoon salt and cook until onions are softened and well browned, 10 to 12 minutes. Stir in coriander and pepper flakes and cook until fragrant, about 30 seconds. Stir in broth, scraping up any browned bits, then stir in chickpeas, sage, and bay leaves.
3. Lock lid in place and close pressure release valve. Select low pressure cook function and cook for 10 minutes. Turn off Instant Pot and let pressure release naturally for 15 minutes. Quick-release any remaining pressure, then carefully remove lid, allowing steam to escape away from you.
4. Discard bay leaves. Stir lemon zest and juice into chickpeas and season with salt and pepper to taste. Sprinkle with parsley. Serve, drizzling individual portions with extra oil.

Per Serving
calories: 190 | fat: 6g | protein: 11g
carbs: 40g | fiber: 1g | sodium: 360mg

Green Bean and Halloumi Cheese Salad

Prep time: 15 minutes | Cook time: 6 minutes | Serves 2

For the Dressing:

¼ cup plain kefir or buttermilk
1 tablespoon olive oil
2 teaspoons freshly squeezed lemon juice
¼ teaspoon onion powder

¼ teaspoon garlic powder
Pinch salt
Pinch freshly ground black pepper

For the Salad:

½ pound (227 g) very fresh green beans, trimmed
2 ounces (57 g) Halloumi cheese, sliced into 2 (½-inch-thick) slices

½ cup cherry or grape tomatoes, halved
¼ cup very thinly sliced sweet onion
2 ounces (57 g) prosciutto, cooked crisp and crumbled

Make the Dressing

1. Combine the kefir or buttermilk, olive oil, lemon juice, onion powder, garlic powder, salt, and pepper in a small bowl and whisk well. Set the dressing aside.

Make the Salad

1. Fill a medium-size pot with about 1 inch of water and add the green beans. Cover and steam them for about 3 to 4 minutes, or just until beans are tender. Do not overcook. Drain beans, rinse them immediately with cold water, and set them aside to cool.
2. Heat a nonstick skillet over medium-high heat and place the slices of Halloumi in the hot pan. After about 2 minutes, check to see if the cheese is golden on the bottom. If it is, flip the slices and cook for another minute or until the second side is golden.
3. Remove cheese from the pan and cut each piece into cubes (about 1-inch square)
4. Place the green beans, halloumi, tomatoes, and sliced onion in a large bowl and toss to combine.
5. Drizzle dressing over the salad and toss well to combine. Sprinkle prosciutto over the top.

Per Serving

calories: 273 | fat: 18g | protein: 15g | carbs: 16g | fiber: 5g | sodium: 506mg

Roasted White Beans with Herb

Prep time: 10 minutes | Cook time: 15 minutes | Serves 4

Olive oil cooking spray
2 (15-ounce / 425-g) cans white beans, or
cannellini beans, drained and rinsed
1 red bell pepper, diced
½ red onion, diced
3 garlic cloves, minced

1 tablespoon olive oil
¼ to ½ teaspoon salt
½ teaspoon black pepper
1 rosemary sprig
1 bay leaf

1. Preheat the air fryer to 360ºF (182ºC). Lightly coat the inside of a 5-cup capacity casserole dish with olive oil cooking spray. (The shape of the casserole dish will depend upon the size of the air fryer, but it needs to be able to hold at least 5 cups.)
2. In a large bowl, combine the beans, bell pepper, onion, garlic, olive oil, salt, and pepper.
3. Pour the bean mixture into the prepared casserole dish, place the rosemary and bay leaf on top, and then place the casserole dish into the air fryer.
4. Roast for 15 minutes.
5. Remove the rosemary and bay leaves, then stir well before serving.

Per Serving
calories: 196 | fat: 5g | protein: 10g | carbs: 30g | fiber: 1g | sodium: 150mg

Butter Beans Casserole with Parsley

Prep time: 10 minutes | Cook time: 30 minutes | Serves 4

Olive oil cooking spray
1 (15-ounce / 425-g) can cooked butter
beans, drained and rinsed
1 cup diced fresh tomatoes
½ tablespoon tomato paste

2 garlic cloves, minced
½ yellow onion, diced
½ teaspoon salt
¼ cup olive oil
¼ cup fresh parsley, chopped

1. Preheat the air fryer to 380ºF (193ºC). Lightly coat the inside of a 5-cup capacity casserole dish with olive oil cooking spray. (The shape of the casserole dish will depend upon the size of the air fryer, but it needs to be able to hold at least 5 cups.)
2. In a large bowl, combine the butter beans, tomatoes, tomato paste, garlic, onion, salt, and olive oil, mixing until all ingredients are combined.
3. Pour the mixture into the prepared casserole dish and top with the chopped parsley.
4. Bake in the air fryer for 15 minutes. Stir well, then return to the air fryer and bake for 15 minutes more.

Per Serving
calories: 212 | fat: 14g | protein: 5g | carbs: 17g | fiber: 1g | sodium: 298mg

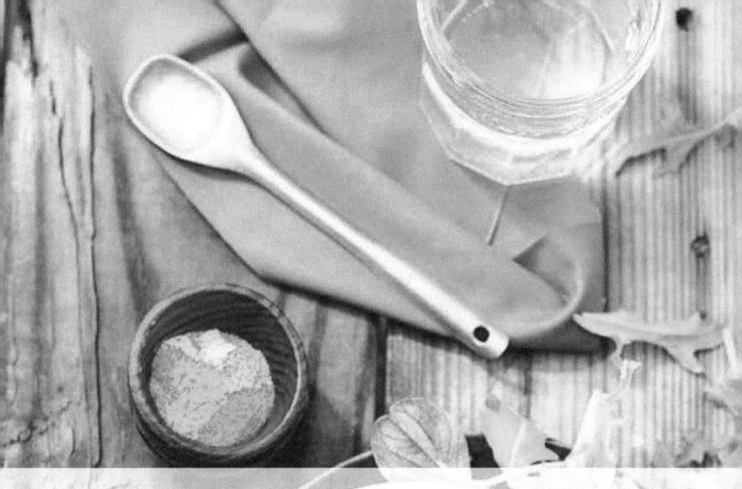

Chapter 13 Grains and Rice

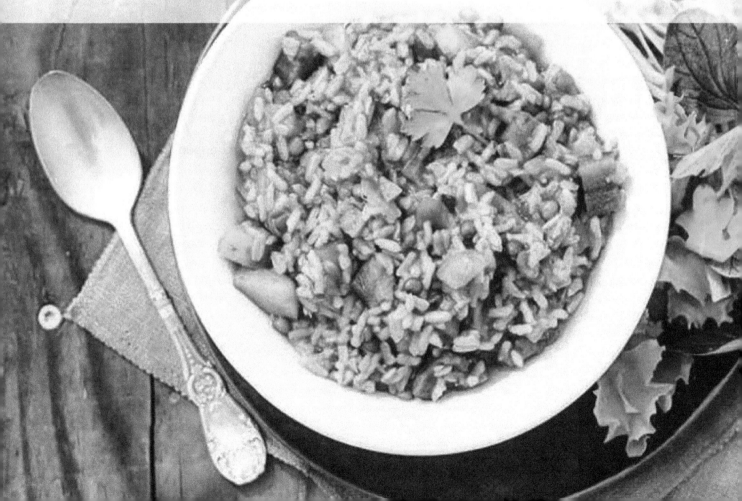

Couscous Confetti Salad

Prep time: 5 minutes | Cook time: 20 minutes | Serves 4 to 6

3 tablespoons extra-virgin olive oil
1 large onion, chopped
2 carrots, chopped
1 cup fresh peas
½ cup golden raisins
1 teaspoon salt
2 cups vegetable broth
2 cups couscous

1. In a medium pot over medium heat, gently toss the olive oil, onions, carrots, peas, and raisins together and let cook for 5 minutes.
2. Add the salt and broth, and stir to combine. Bring to a boil, and let ingredients boil for 5 minutes.
3. Add the couscous. Stir, turn the heat to low, cover, and let cook for 10 minutes. Fluff with a fork and serve.

Per Serving

calories: 511 | fat: 12g | protein: 14g
carbs: 92g | fiber: 7g | sodium: 504mg

Rustic Lentil-Rice Pilaf

Prep time: 5 minutes | Cook time: 50 minutes | Serves 6

¼ cup extra-virgin olive oil
1 large onion, chopped
6 cups water
1 teaspoon ground
cumin
1 teaspoon salt
2 cups brown lentils, picked over and rinsed
1 cup basmati rice

1. In a medium pot over medium heat, cook the olive oil and onions for 7 to 10 minutes until the edges are browned.
2. Turn the heat to high, add the water, cumin, and salt, and bring this mixture to a boil, boiling for about 3 minutes.
3. Add the lentils and turn the heat to medium-low. Cover the pot and cook for 20 minutes, stirring occasionally.
4. Stir in the rice and cover; cook for an additional 20 minutes.
5. Fluff the rice with a fork and serve warm.

Per Serving

calories: 397 | fat: 11g | protein: 18g
carbs: 60g | fiber: 18g | sodium: 396mg

Bulgur Pilaf with Garbanzos

Prep time: 5 minutes | Cook time: 20 minutes | Serves 4 to 6

3 tablespoons extra-virgin olive oil
1 large onion, chopped
1 (16-ounce / 454-g) can garbanzo beans, rinsed and drained
2 cups bulgur wheat, rinsed and drained
1½ teaspoons salt
½ teaspoon cinnamon
4 cups water

1. In a large pot over medium heat, cook the olive oil and onion for 5 minutes.
2. Add the garbanzo beans and cook for another 5 minutes.
3. Add the bulgur, salt, cinnamon, and water and stir to combine. Cover the pot, turn the heat to low, and cook for 10 minutes.
4. When the cooking is done, fluff the pilaf with a fork. Cover and let sit for another 5 minutes.

Per Serving

calories: 462 | fat: 13g | protein: 15g
carbs: 76g | fiber: 19g | sodium: 890mg

Simple Spanish Rice

Prep time: 10 minutes | Cook time: 20 minutes | Serves 4

2 tablespoons extra-virgin olive oil
1 medium onion, finely chopped
1 large tomato, finely diced
2 tablespoons tomato
paste
1 teaspoon smoked paprika
1 teaspoon salt
1½ cups basmati rice
3 cups water

1. In a medium pot over medium heat, cook the olive oil, onion, and tomato for 3 minutes.
2. Stir in the tomato paste, paprika, salt, and rice. Cook for 1 minute.
3. Add the water, cover the pot, and turn the heat to low. Cook for 12 minutes.
4. Gently toss the rice, cover, and cook for another 3 minutes.

Per Serving

calories: 328 | fat: 7g | protein: 6g
carbs: 60g | fiber: 2g | sodium: 651mg

Lentil Bulgur Pilaf

Prep time: 10 minutes | Cook time: 50 minutes | Serves 6

½ cup extra-virgin olive oil
4 large onions, chopped
2 teaspoons salt, divided
6 cups water
2 cups brown lentils, picked over and rinsed
1 teaspoon freshly ground black pepper
1 cup bulgur wheat

1. In a large pot over medium heat, cook and stir the olive oil, onions, and 1 teaspoon of salt for 12 to 15 minutes, until the onions are a medium brown/golden color.
2. Put half of the cooked onions in a bowl.
3. Add the water, remaining 1 teaspoon of salt, and lentils to the remaining onions. Stir. Cover and cook for 30 minutes.
4. Stir in the black pepper and bulgur, cover, and cook for 5 minutes. Fluff with a fork, cover, and let stand for another 5 minutes.
5. Spoon the lentils and bulgur onto a serving plate and top with the reserved onions. Serve warm.

Per Serving
calories: 479 | fat: 20g | protein: 20g
carbs: 60g | fiber: 24g | sodium: 789mg

Creamy Parmesan Garlic Polenta

Prep time: 5 minutes | Cook time: 30 minutes | Serves 4

4 tablespoons (½ stick) unsalted butter, divided (optional)
1 tablespoon garlic, finely chopped
4 cups water
1 teaspoon salt
1 cup polenta
¾ cup Parmesan cheese, divided

1. In a large pot over medium heat, cook 3 tablespoons of butter (if desired) and the garlic for 2 minutes.
2. Add the water and salt, and bring to a boil. Add the polenta and immediately whisk until it starts to thicken, about 3 minutes. Turn the heat to low, cover, and cook for 25 minutes, whisking every 5 minutes.

3. Using a wooden spoon, stir in ½ cup of the Parmesan cheese.
4. To serve, pour the polenta into a large serving bowl. Sprinkle the top with the remaining 1 tablespoon butter (if desired) and ¼ cup of remaining Parmesan cheese. Serve warm.

Per Serving
calories: 297 | fat: 16g | protein: 9g
carbs: 28g | fiber: 2g | sodium: 838mg

Mushroom Parmesan Risotto

Prep time: 10 minutes | Cook time: 30 minutes | Serves 4

6 cups vegetable broth
3 tablespoons extra-virgin olive oil, divided
1 pound (454 g) cremini mushrooms, cleaned and sliced
1 medium onion, finely chopped
2 cloves garlic, minced
1½ cups Arborio rice
1 teaspoon salt
½ cup freshly grated Parmesan cheese
½ teaspoon freshly ground black pepper

1. In a saucepan over medium heat, bring the broth to a low simmer.
2. In a large skillet over medium heat, cook 1 tablespoon olive oil and the sliced mushrooms for 5 to 7 minutes. Set cooked mushrooms aside.
3. In the same skillet over medium heat, add the 2 remaining tablespoons of olive oil, onion, and garlic. Cook for 3 minutes.
4. Add the rice, salt, and 1 cup of broth to the skillet. Stir the ingredients together and cook over low heat until most of the liquid is absorbed. Continue adding ½ cup of broth at a time, stirring until it is absorbed. Repeat until all of the broth is used up.
5. With the final addition of broth, add the cooked mushrooms, Parmesan cheese, and black pepper. Cook for 2 more minutes. Serve immediately.

Per Serving
calories: 410 | fat: 12g | protein: 11g
carbs: 65g | fiber: 3g | sodium: 2086mg

Wild Mushroom Farrotto with Parmesan

Prep time: 15 minutes | Cook time: 7 minutes | Serves 4

1½ cups whole farro
3 tablespoons extra-virgin olive oil, divided, plus extra for drizzling
12 ounces (340 g) cremini or white mushrooms, trimmed and sliced thin
½ onion, chopped fine
½ teaspoon table salt
¼ teaspoon pepper
1 garlic clove, minced
¼ ounce (7 g) dried porcini mushrooms, rinsed and chopped
fine
2 teaspoons minced fresh thyme or ½ teaspoon dried
¼ cup dry white wine
2½ cups chicken or vegetable broth, plus extra as needed
2 ounces (57 g) Parmesan cheese, grated, plus extra for serving
2 teaspoons lemon juice
½ cup chopped fresh parsley

1. Pulse farro in blender until about half of grains are broken into smaller pieces, about 6 pulses.
2. Using highest sauté function, heat 2 tablespoons oil in Instant Pot until shimmering. Add cremini mushrooms, onion, salt, and pepper, partially cover, and cook until mushrooms are softened and have released their liquid, about 5 minutes. Stir in farro, garlic, porcini mushrooms, and thyme and cook until fragrant, about 1 minute. Stir in wine and cook until nearly evaporated, about 30 seconds. Stir in broth.
3. Lock lid in place and close pressure release valve. Select high pressure cook function and cook for 12 minutes. Turn off Instant Pot and quick-release pressure. Carefully remove lid, allowing steam to escape away from you.
4. If necessary adjust consistency with extra hot broth, or continue to cook farrotto, using highest sauté function, stirring frequently, until proper consistency is achieved. (Farrotto should be slightly thickened, and spoon dragged along bottom of multicooker should leave trail that quickly fills in.) Add Parmesan and remaining 1 tablespoon oil and stir vigorously until farrotto becomes creamy. Stir in lemon juice and season with salt and pepper to taste. Sprinkle individual portions with parsley and extra Parmesan, and drizzle with extra oil before serving.

Per Serving
calories: 280 | fat: 9g | protein: 13g
carbs: 35g | fiber: 3g | sodium: 630mg

Moroccan-Style Brown Rice and Chickpea

Prep time: 15 minutes | Cook time: 45 minutes | Serves 6

Olive oil cooking spray
1 cup long-grain brown rice
2¼ cups chicken stock
1 (15½-ounce / 439-g) can chickpeas, drained and rinsed
½ cup diced carrot
½ cup green peas
1 teaspoon ground cumin
½ teaspoon ground
turmeric
½ teaspoon ground ginger
½ teaspoon onion powder
½ teaspoon salt
¼ teaspoon ground cinnamon
¼ teaspoon garlic powder
¼ teaspoon black pepper
Fresh parsley, for garnish

1. Preheat the air fryer to 380ºF (193ºC). Lightly coat the inside of a 5-cup capacity casserole dish with olive oil cooking spray. (The shape of the casserole dish will depend upon the size of the air fryer, but it needs to be able to hold at least 5 cups.)
2. In the casserole dish, combine the rice, stock, chickpeas, carrot, peas, cumin, turmeric, ginger, onion powder, salt, cinnamon, garlic powder, and black pepper. Stir well to combine.
3. Cover loosely with aluminum foil.
4. Place the covered casserole dish into the air fryer and bake for 20 minutes. Remove from the air fryer and stir well.
5. Place the casserole back into the air fryer, uncovered, and bake for 25 minutes more.
6. Fluff with a spoon and sprinkle with fresh chopped parsley before serving.

Per Serving
calories: 204 | fat: 1g | protein: 7g
carbs: 40g | fiber: 4g | sodium: 623mg

Freekeh Pilaf with Dates and Pistachios

Prep time: 10 minutes | Cook time: 10 minutes | Serves 4 to 6

2 tablespoons extra-virgin olive oil, plus extra for drizzling
1 shallot, minced
1½ teaspoons grated fresh ginger
¼ teaspoon ground coriander
¼ teaspoon ground cumin
Salt and pepper, to taste

1¾ cups water
1½ cups cracked freekeh, rinsed
3 ounces (85 g) pitted dates, chopped
¼ cup shelled pistachios, toasted and coarsely chopped
1½ tablespoons lemon juice
¼ cup chopped fresh mint

1. Set the Instant Pot to Sauté mode and heat the olive oil until shimmering.
2. Add the shallot, ginger, coriander, cumin, salt, and pepper to the pot and cook for about 2 minutes, or until the shallot is softened. Stir in the water and freekeh.
3. Secure the lid. Select the Manual mode and set the cooking time for 4 minutes at High Pressure. Once cooking is complete, do a quick pressure release. Carefully open the lid.
4. Add the dates, pistachios and lemon juice and gently fluff the freekeh with a fork to combine. Season to taste with salt and pepper.
5. Transfer to a serving dish and sprinkle with the mint. Serve drizzled with extra olive oil.

Per Serving
calories: 280 | fat: 8g | protein: 8g
carbs: 46g | fiber: 9g | sodium: 200mg

Farro Risotto with Fresh Sage

Prep time: 10 minutes | Cook time: 35 minutes | Serves 6

Olive oil cooking spray
1½ cups uncooked farro
2 ½ cups chicken broth
1 cup tomato sauce
1 yellow onion, diced
3 garlic cloves,

minced
1 tablespoon fresh sage, chopped
½ teaspoon salt
2 tablespoons olive oil
1 cup Parmesan cheese, grated, divided

1. Preheat the air fryer to 380ºF (193ºC). Lightly coat the inside of a 5-cup capacity casserole dish with olive oil cooking spray. (The shape of the casserole dish will depend upon the size of the air fryer, but it needs to be able to hold at least 5 cups.)
2. In a large bowl, combine the farro, broth, tomato sauce, onion, garlic, sage, salt, olive oil, and ½ cup of the Parmesan.
3. Pour the farro mixture into the prepared casserole dish and cover with aluminum foil.
4. Bake for 20 minutes, then uncover and stir. Sprinkle the remaining ½ cup Parmesan over the top and bake for 15 minutes more.
5. Stir well before serving.

Per Serving
calories: 284 | fat: 9g | protein: 12g
carbs: 40g | fiber: 3g | sodium: 564mg

Toasted Barley and Almond Pilaf

Prep time: 10 minutes | Cook time: 5 minutes | Serves 2

1 tablespoon olive oil
1 garlic clove, minced
3 scallions, minced
2 ounces (57 g) mushrooms, sliced
¼ cup sliced almonds
½ cup uncooked pearled barley

1½ cups low-sodium chicken stock
½ teaspoon dried thyme
1 tablespoon fresh minced parsley
Salt, to taste

1. Heat the oil in a saucepan over medium-high heat. Add the garlic, scallions, mushrooms, and almonds, and sauté for 3 minutes.
2. Add the barley and cook, stirring, for 1 minute to toast it.
3. Add the chicken stock and thyme and bring the mixture to a boil.
4. Cover and reduce the heat to low. Simmer the barley for 30 minutes, or until the liquid is absorbed and the barley is tender.
5. Sprinkle with fresh parsley and season with salt before serving.

Per Serving
calories: 333 | fat: 13g | protein: 10g
carbs: 46g | fiber: 9g | sodium: 141mg

Spanish Chicken and Rice

Prep time: 15 minutes | Cook time: 30 minutes | Serves 2

2 teaspoons smoked paprika
2 teaspoons ground cumin
1½ teaspoons garlic salt
¾ teaspoon chili powder
¼ teaspoon dried oregano
1 lemon
2 boneless, skinless chicken breasts
3 tablespoons extra-virgin olive oil, divided
2 large shallots, diced
1 cup uncooked white rice
2 cups vegetable stock
1 cup broccoli florets
¹/₃ cup chopped parsley

1. In a small bowl, whisk together the paprika, cumin, garlic salt, chili powder, and oregano. Divide in half and set aside. Into another small bowl, juice the lemon and set aside.
2. Put the chicken in a medium bowl. Coat the chicken with 2 tablespoons of olive oil and rub with half of the seasoning mix.
3. In a large pan, heat the remaining 1 tablespoon of olive oil and cook the chicken for 2 to 3 minutes on each side, until just browned but not cooked through.
4. Add shallots to the same pan and cook until translucent, then add the rice and cook for 1 more minute to toast. Add the vegetable stock, lemon juice, and the remaining seasoning mix and stir to combine. Return the chicken to the pan on top of the rice. Cover and cook for 15 minutes.
5. Uncover and add the broccoli florets. Cover and cook an additional 5 minutes, until the liquid is absorbed, rice is tender, and chicken is cooked through.
6. Top with freshly chopped parsley and serve immediately.

Per Serving
calories: 750 | fat: 25g | protein: 36g
carbs: 101g | fiber: 7g | sodium: 1823mg

Buckwheat Groats with Root Vegetables

Prep time: 15 minutes | Cook time: 40 minutes | Serves 6

Olive oil cooking spray
2 large potatoes, cubed
2 carrots, sliced
1 small rutabaga, cubed
2 celery stalks, chopped
½ teaspoon smoked paprika
¼ cup plus 1
tablespoon olive oil, divided
2 rosemary sprigs
1 cup buckwheat groats
2 cups vegetable broth
2 garlic cloves, minced
½ yellow onion, chopped
1 teaspoon salt

1. Preheat the air fryer to 380ºF (193ºC). Lightly coat the inside of a 5-cup capacity casserole dish with olive oil cooking spray. (The shape of the casserole dish will depend upon the size of the air fryer, but it needs to be able to hold at least 5 cups.)
2. In a large bowl, toss the potatoes, carrots, rutabaga, and celery with the paprika and ¼ cup olive oil.
3. Pour the vegetable mixture into the prepared casserole dish and top with the rosemary sprigs. Place the casserole dish into the air fryer and bake for 15 minutes.
4. While the vegetables are cooking, rinse and drain the buckwheat groats.
5. In a medium saucepan over medium-high heat, combine the groats, vegetable broth, garlic, onion, and salt with the remaining 1 tablespoon olive oil. Bring the mixture to a boil, then reduce the heat to low, cover, and cook for 10 to 12 minutes.
6. Remove the casserole dish from the air fryer. Remove the rosemary sprigs and discard. Pour the cooked buckwheat into the dish with the vegetables and stir to combine. Cover with aluminum foil and bake for an additional 15 minutes.
7. Stir before serving.

Per Serving
calories: 344 | fat: 12g | protein: 8g
carbs: 50g | fiber: 7g | sodium: 876mg

Mushroom Barley Pilaf

Prep time: 5 minutes | Cook time: 37 minutes | Serves 4

Olive oil cooking spray
2 tablespoons olive oil
8 ounces (227 g) button mushrooms, diced
½ yellow onion, diced
2 garlic cloves, minced
1 cup pearl barley
2 cups vegetable broth
1 tablespoon fresh thyme, chopped
½ teaspoon salt
¼ teaspoon smoked paprika
Fresh parsley, for garnish

1. Preheat the air fryer to 380ºF (193ºC). Lightly coat the inside of a 5-cup capacity casserole dish with olive oil cooking spray. (The shape of the casserole dish will depend upon the size of the air fryer, but it needs to be able to hold at least 5 cups.)
2. In a large skillet, heat the olive oil over medium heat. Add the mushrooms and onion and cook, stirring occasionally, for 5 minutes, or until the mushrooms begin to brown.
3. Add the garlic and cook for an additional 2 minutes. Transfer the vegetables to a large bowl.
4. Add the barley, broth, thyme, salt, and paprika.
5. Pour the barley-and-vegetable mixture into the prepared casserole dish, and place the dish into the air fryer. Bake for 15 minutes.
6. Stir the barley mixture. Reduce the heat to 360ºF (182ºC), then return the barley to the air fryer and bake for 15 minutes more.
7. Remove from the air fryer and let sit for 5 minutes before fluffing with a fork and topping with fresh parsley.

Per Serving
calories: 263 | fat: 8g | protein: 7g
carbs: 44g | fiber: 9g | sodium: 576mg

Mediterranean Lentils and Brown Rice

Prep time: 15 minutes | Cook time: 23 minutes | Serves 4

2¼ cups low-sodium or no-salt-added vegetable broth
½ cup uncooked brown or green lentils
½ cup uncooked instant brown rice
½ cup diced carrots
½ cup diced celery
1 (2¼-ounce / 64-g) can sliced olives, drained
¼ cup diced red
onion
¼ cup chopped fresh curly-leaf parsley
1½ tablespoons extra-virgin olive oil
1 tablespoon freshly squeezed lemon juice
1 garlic clove, minced
¼ teaspoon kosher or sea salt
¼ teaspoon freshly ground black pepper

1. In a medium saucepan over high heat, bring the broth and lentils to a boil, cover, and lower the heat to medium-low. Cook for 8 minutes.
2. Raise the heat to medium, and stir in the rice. Cover the pot and cook the mixture for 15 minutes, or until the liquid is absorbed. Remove the pot from the heat and let it sit, covered, for 1 minute, then stir.
3. While the lentils and rice are cooking, mix together the carrots, celery, olives, onion, and parsley in a large serving bowl.
4. In a small bowl, whisk together the oil, lemon juice, garlic, salt, and pepper. Set aside.
5. When the lentils and rice are cooked, add them to the serving bowl. Pour the dressing on top, and mix everything together. Serve warm or cold, or store in a sealed container in the refrigerator for up to 7 days.

Per Serving
calories: 170 | fat: 5g | protein: 5g
carbs: 25g | fiber: 2g | sodium: 566mg

Brown Rice Bowls with Roasted Vegetables

Prep time: 15 minutes | Cook time: 20 minutes | Serves 4

Nonstick cooking spray
2 cups broccoli florets
2 cups cauliflower florets
1 (15-ounce / 425-g) can chickpeas, drained and rinsed
1 cup carrots sliced 1 inch thick
2 to 3 tablespoons
extra-virgin olive oil, divided
Salt and freshly ground black pepper, to taste
2 to 3 tablespoons sesame seeds, for garnish
2 cups cooked brown rice

Dressing:
3 to 4 tablespoons tahini
2 tablespoons honey
1 lemon, juiced
1 garlic clove, minced
Salt and freshly ground black pepper, to taste

1. Preheat the oven to 400ºF (205ºC). Spray two baking sheets with cooking spray.
2. Cover the first baking sheet with the broccoli and cauliflower and the second with the chickpeas and carrots. Toss each sheet with half of the oil and season with salt and pepper before placing in oven.
3. Cook the carrots and chickpeas for 10 minutes, leaving the carrots still just crisp, and the broccoli and cauliflower for 20 minutes, until tender. Stir each halfway through cooking.
4. To make the dressing, in a small bowl, mix the tahini, honey, lemon juice, and garlic. Season with salt and pepper and set aside.
5. Divide the rice into individual bowls, then layer with vegetables and drizzle dressing over the dish.

Per Serving
calories: 454 | fat: 18g | protein: 12g
carbs: 62g | fiber: 11g | sodium: 61mg

Pearl Barley Risotto with Parmesan Cheese

Prep time: 5 minutes | Cook time: 20 minutes | Serves 6

4 cups low-sodium or no-salt-added vegetable broth
1 tablespoon extra-virgin olive oil
1 cup chopped yellow onion
2 cups uncooked pearl barley
½ cup dry white wine
1 cup freshly grated Parmesan cheese, divided
¼ teaspoon kosher or sea salt
¼ teaspoon freshly ground black pepper
Fresh chopped chives and lemon wedges, for serving (optional)

1. Pour the broth into a medium saucepan and bring to a simmer.
2. Heat the olive oil in a large stockpot over medium-high heat. Add the onion and cook for about 4 minutes, stirring occasionally.
3. Add the barley and cook for 2 minutes, stirring, or until the barley is toasted. Pour in the wine and cook for about 1 minute, or until most of the liquid evaporates. Add 1 cup of the warm broth into the pot and cook, stirring, for about 2 minutes, or until most of the liquid is absorbed.
4. Add the remaining broth, 1 cup at a time, cooking until each cup is absorbed (about 2 minutes each time) before adding the next. The last addition of broth will take a bit longer to absorb, about 4 minutes.
5. Remove the pot from the heat, and stir in ½ cup of the cheese, and the salt and pepper.
6. Serve with the remaining ½ cup of the cheese on the side, along with the chives and lemon wedges (if desired).

Per Serving
calories: 421 | fat: 11g | protein: 15g
carbs: 67g | fiber: 11g | sodium: 641mg

Israeli Couscous with Asparagus

Prep time: 5 minutes | Cook time: 25 minutes | Serves 6

1½ pounds (680 g) asparagus spears, ends trimmed and stalks chopped into 1-inch pieces	1 (8-ounce / 227-g) box uncooked whole-wheat or regular Israeli couscous (about 1⅓ cups)
1 garlic clove, minced	¼ teaspoon kosher salt
1 tablespoon extra-virgin olive oil	1 cup garlic-and-herb goat cheese, at room temperature
¼ teaspoon freshly ground black pepper	
1¾ cups water	

1. Preheat the oven to 425ºF (220ºC).
2. In a large bowl, stir together the asparagus, garlic, oil, and pepper. Spread the asparagus on a large, rimmed baking sheet and roast for 10 minutes, stirring a few times. Remove the pan from the oven, and spoon the asparagus into a large serving bowl. Set aside.
3. While the asparagus is roasting, bring the water to a boil in a medium saucepan. Add the couscous and season with salt, stirring well.
4. Reduce the heat to medium-low. Cover and cook for 12 minutes, or until the water is absorbed.
5. Pour the hot couscous into the bowl with the asparagus. Add the goat cheese and mix thoroughly until completely melted.
6. Serve immediately.

Per Serving

calories: 103 | fat: 2g | protein: 6g
carbs: 18g | fiber: 5g | sodium: 343mg

Quinoa with Baby Potatoes and Broccoli

Prep time: 5 minutes | Cook time: 10 minutes | Serves 4

2 tablespoons olive oil	2 cups cooked quinoa
1 cup baby potatoes, cut in half	Zest of 1 lemon
1 cup broccoli florets	Sea salt and freshly ground pepper, to taste

1. Heat the olive oil in a large skillet over medium heat until shimmering.

2. Add the potatoes and cook for about 6 to 7 minutes, or until softened and golden brown. Add the broccoli and cook for about 3 minutes, or until tender.
3. Remove from the heat and add the quinoa and lemon zest. Season with salt and pepper to taste, then serve.

Per Serving

calories: 205 | fat: 8g | protein: 5g
carbs: 27g | fiber: 3g | sodium: 158mg

Bulgur with Za'Atar, Chickpeas, and Spinach

Prep time: 10 minutes | Cook time: 7 minutes | Serves 4 to 6

3 tablespoons extra-virgin olive oil, divided	bulgur, rinsed
	1 (15-ounce / 425-g) can chickpeas, rinsed
1 onion, chopped fine	1½ cups water
½ teaspoon table salt	5 ounces (142 g) baby spinach, chopped
3 garlic cloves, minced	
2 tablespoons za'atar, divided	1 tablespoon lemon juice, plus lemon wedges for serving
1 cup medium-grind	

1. Using highest sauté function, heat 2 tablespoons oil in Instant Pot until shimmering. Add onion and salt and cook until onion is softened, about 5 minutes. Stir in garlic and 1 tablespoon za'atar and cook until fragrant, about 30 seconds. Stir in bulgur, chickpeas, and water.
2. Lock lid in place and close pressure release valve. Select high pressure cook function and cook for 1 minute. Turn off Instant Pot and quick-release pressure. Carefully remove lid, allowing steam to escape away from you.
3. Gently fluff bulgur with fork. Lay clean dish towel over pot, replace lid, and let sit for 5 minutes. Add spinach, lemon juice, remaining 1 tablespoon za'atar, and remaining 1 tablespoon oil and gently toss to combine. Season with salt and pepper to taste. Serve with lemon wedges.

Per Serving

calories: 200 | fat: 8g | protein: 6g
carbs: 28g | fiber: 6g | sodium: 320mg

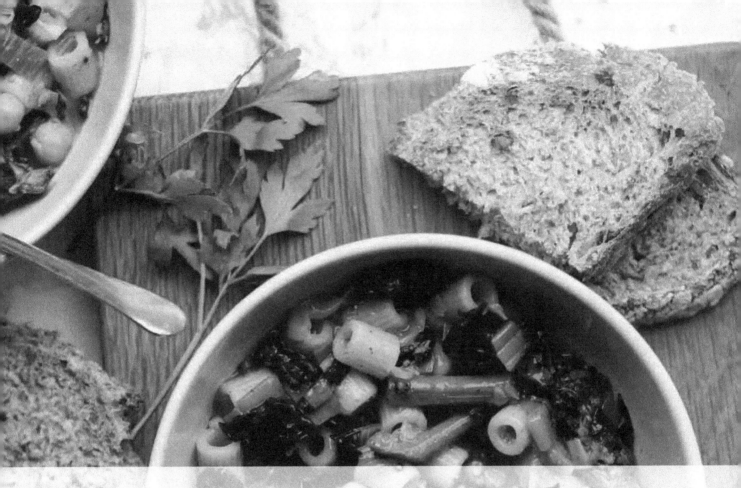
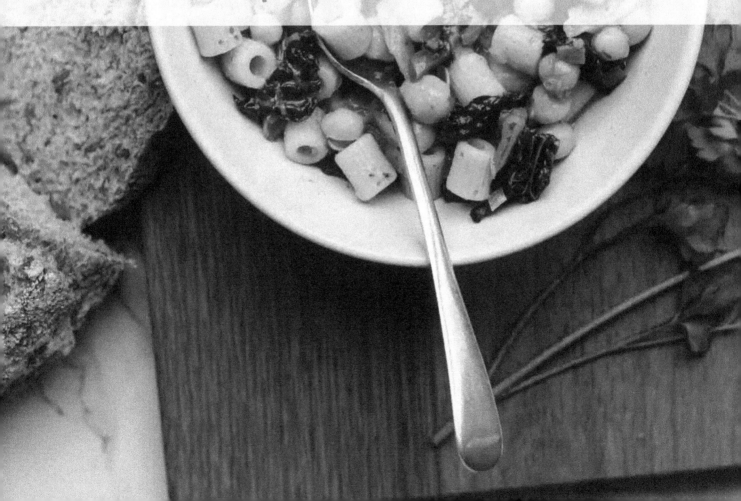

Chapter 14 Pasta

Spaghetti with Pine Nuts and Cheese

Prep time: 10 minutes | Cook time: 11 minutes | Serves 4 to 6

8 ounces (227 g) spaghetti
4 tablespoons almond butter
1 teaspoon freshly

ground black pepper
½ cup pine nuts
1 cup fresh grated Parmesan cheese, divided

1. Bring a large pot of salted water to a boil. Add the pasta and cook for 8 minutes.
2. In a large saucepan over medium heat, combine the butter, black pepper, and pine nuts. Cook for 2 to 3 minutes, or until the pine nuts are lightly toasted.
3. Reserve ½ cup of the pasta water. Drain the pasta and place it into the pan with the pine nuts.
4. Add ¾ cup of the Parmesan cheese and the reserved pasta water to the pasta and toss everything together to evenly coat the pasta.
5. Transfer the pasta to a serving dish and top with the remaining ¼ cup of the Parmesan cheese. Serve immediately.

Per Serving
calories: 542 | fat: 32g | protein: 20g
carbs: 46g | fiber: 2g | sodium: 552mg

Garlic Shrimp Fettuccine

Prep time: 10 minutes | Cook time: 15 minutes | Serves 4 to 6

8 ounces (227 g) fettuccine pasta
¼ cup extra-virgin olive oil
3 tablespoons garlic, minced
1 pound (454 g) large shrimp, peeled

and deveined
⅓ cup lemon juice
1 tablespoon lemon zest
½ teaspoon salt
½ teaspoon freshly ground black pepper

1. Bring a large pot of salted water to a boil. Add the fettuccine and cook for 8 minutes. Reserve ½ cup of the cooking liquid and drain the pasta.
2. In a large saucepan over medium heat, heat the olive oil. Add the garlic and sauté for 1 minute.

3. Add the shrimp to the saucepan and cook each side for 3 minutes. Remove the shrimp from the pan and set aside.
4. Add the remaining ingredients to the saucepan. Stir in the cooking liquid. Add the pasta and toss together to evenly coat the pasta.
5. Transfer the pasta to a serving dish and serve topped with the cooked shrimp.

Per Serving
calories: 485 | fat: 17g | protein: 33g
carbs: 50g | fiber: 4g | sodium: 407mg

Simple Pesto Pasta

Prep time: 10 minutes | Cook time: 8 minutes | Serves 4 to 6

1 pound (454 g) spaghetti
4 cups fresh basil leaves, stems removed
3 cloves garlic
1 teaspoon salt
½ teaspoon freshly

ground black pepper
½ cup toasted pine nuts
¼ cup lemon juice
½ cup grated Parmesan cheese
1 cup extra-virgin olive oil

1. Bring a large pot of salted water to a boil. Add the spaghetti to the pot and cook for 8 minutes.
2. In a food processor, place the remaining ingredients, except for the olive oil, and pulse.
3. While the processor is running, slowly drizzle the olive oil through the top opening. Process until all the olive oil has been added.
4. Reserve ½ cup of the cooking liquid. Drain the pasta and put it into a large bowl. Add the pesto and cooking liquid to the bowl of pasta and toss everything together.
5. Serve immediately.

Per Serving
calories: 1067 | fat: 72g | protein: 23g
carbs: 91g | fiber: 6g | sodium: 817mg

Whole-Wheat Fusilli with Chickpea Sauce

Prep time: 15 minutes | Cook time: 15 minutes | Serves 4

¼ cup extra-virgin olive oil
½ large shallot, chopped
5 garlic cloves, thinly sliced
1 (15-ounce / 425-g) can chickpeas, drained and rinsed, reserving ½ cup canning liquid
Pinch red pepper flakes
1 cup whole-grain
fusilli pasta
¼ teaspoon salt
⅛ teaspoon freshly ground black pepper
¼ cup shaved fresh Parmesan cheese
¼ cup chopped fresh basil
2 teaspoons dried parsley
1 teaspoon dried oregano
Red pepper flakes

1. In a medium pan, heat the oil over medium heat, and sauté the shallot and garlic for 3 to 5 minutes, until the garlic is golden. Add ¾ of the chickpeas plus 2 tablespoons of liquid from the can, and bring to a simmer.
2. Remove from the heat, transfer into a standard blender, and blend until smooth. At this point, add the remaining chickpeas. Add more reserved chickpea liquid if it becomes thick.
3. Bring a large pot of salted water to a boil and cook pasta until al dente, about 8 minutes. Reserve ½ cup of the pasta water, drain the pasta, and return it to the pot.
4. Add the chickpea sauce to the hot pasta and add up to ¼ cup of the pasta water. You may need to add more pasta water to reach your desired consistency.
5. Place the pasta pot over medium heat and mix occasionally until the sauce thickens. Season with salt and pepper.
6. Serve, garnished with Parmesan, basil, parsley, oregano, and red pepper flakes.

Per Serving (1 cup pasta)
calories: 310 | fat: 16g | protein: 10g
carbs: 33g | fiber: 6g | sodium: 243mg

Bow Ties with Zucchini

Prep time: 10 minutes | Cook time: 32 minutes | Serves 4

3 tablespoons extra-virgin olive oil
2 garlic cloves, minced
3 large or 4 medium zucchini, diced
½ teaspoon freshly ground black pepper
¼ teaspoon kosher or sea salt
½ cup 2% milk
¼ teaspoon ground nutmeg
8 ounces (227 g) uncooked farfalle (bow ties) or other small pasta shape
½ cup grated Parmesan or Romano cheese
1 tablespoon freshly squeezed lemon juice

1. In a large skillet over medium heat, heat the oil. Add the garlic and cook for 1 minute, stirring frequently. Add the zucchini, pepper, and salt. Stir well, cover, and cook for 15 minutes, stirring once or twice.
2. In a small, microwave-safe bowl, warm the milk in the microwave on high for 30 seconds. Stir the milk and nutmeg into the skillet and cook uncovered for another 5 minutes, stirring occasionally.
3. While the zucchini is cooking, in a large stockpot, cook the pasta according to the package directions.
4. Drain the pasta in a colander, saving about 2 tablespoons of pasta water. Add the pasta and pasta water to the skillet. Mix everything together and remove from the heat. Stir in the cheese and lemon juice and serve.

Per Serving
calories: 190 | fat: 9g | protein: 7g
carbs: 20g | fiber: 2g | sodium: 475mg

Linguine with Artichokes and Peas

Prep time: 10 minutes | Cook time: 5 minutes | Serves 4 to 6

1 pound (454 g) linguine
5 cups water, plus extra as needed
1 tablespoon extra-virgin olive oil
1 teaspoon table salt
1 cup jarred whole baby artichokes packed in water, quartered
1 cup frozen peas, thawed
4 ounces (113 g) finely grated Pecorino Romano, plus extra for serving
½ teaspoon pepper
2 teaspoons grated lemon zest
2 tablespoons chopped fresh tarragon

1. Loosely wrap half of pasta in dish towel, then press bundle against corner of counter to break noodles into 6-inch lengths; repeat with remaining pasta.
2. Add pasta, water, oil, and salt to Instant Pot, making sure pasta is completely submerged. Lock lid in place and close pressure release valve. Select high pressure cook function and cook for 4 minutes. Turn off Instant Pot and quick-release pressure. Carefully remove lid, allowing steam to escape away from you.
3. Stir artichokes and peas into pasta, cover, and let sit until heated through, about 3 minutes. Gently stir in Pecorino and pepper until cheese is melted and fully combined, 1 to 2 minutes. Adjust consistency with extra hot water as needed. Stir in lemon zest and tarragon, and season with salt and pepper to taste. Serve, passing extra Pecorino separately.

Per Serving
calories: 390 | fat: 7g | protein: 17g
carbs: 59g | fiber: 3g | sodium: 680mg

Rigatoni with Pancetta and Veggie

Prep time: 15 minutes | Cook time: 22 minutes | Serves 4 to 6

4 ounces (113 g) pancetta, chopped fine
1 onion, chopped fine
¼ teaspoon table salt
3 garlic cloves, minced
2 anchovy fillets, rinsed, patted dry, and minced
2 teaspoons fennel seeds, lightly cracked
¼ teaspoon red pepper flakes
1 (28-ounce / 794-g) can diced tomatoes
2 cups chicken broth
1½ cups water
1 pound (454 g) rigatoni
¼ cup grated Pecorino Romano cheese, plus extra for serving
2 tablespoons minced fresh parsley

1. Using highest sauté function, cook pancetta in Instant Pot, stirring often, until browned and fat is well rendered, 6 to 10 minutes. Using slotted spoon, transfer pancetta to paper towel–lined plate; set aside for serving.
2. Add onion and salt to fat left in pot and cook, using highest sauté function, until onion is softened, about 5 minutes. Stir in garlic, anchovies, fennel seeds, and pepper flakes and cook until fragrant, about 1 minute. Stir in tomatoes and their juice, broth, and water, scraping up any browned bits, then stir in pasta.
3. Lock lid in place and close pressure release valve. Select high pressure cook function and cook for 5 minutes. Turn off Instant Pot and quick-release pressure. Carefully remove lid, allowing steam to escape away from you.
4. Stir in Pecorino and season with salt and pepper to taste. Transfer to serving dish and let sit until sauce thickens slightly, about 5 minutes. Sprinkle with parsley and reserved pancetta. Serve, passing extra Pecorino separately.

Per Serving
calories: 400 | fat: 7g | protein: 17g
carbs: 64g | fiber: 5g | sodium: 1020mg

Orecchiette with Italian Sausage and Broccoli

Prep time: 10 minutes | Cook time: 13 minutes | Serves 4 to 6

2 tablespoons extra-virgin olive oil, divided
1 pound (454 g) broccoli rabe, trimmed and cut into 1½-inch pieces
¼ teaspoon table salt
8 ounces (227 g) hot or sweet Italian sausage, casings removed
6 garlic cloves, minced
¼ teaspoon red pepper flakes
¼ cup dry white wine
4½ cups chicken broth
1 pound (454 g) orecchiette
2 ounces (57 g) Parmesan cheese, grated, plus extra for serving

1. Using highest sauté function, heat 1 tablespoon oil in Instant Pot until shimmering. Add broccoli rabe and salt, partially cover, and cook, stirring occasionally, until broccoli rabe is softened, 3 to 5 minutes. Using slotted spoon, transfer broccoli rabe to bowl; set aside.
2. Add sausage and remaining 1 tablespoon oil to now-empty pot. Using highest sauté function, cook sausage, breaking up meat with wooden spoon, until lightly browned, about 5 minutes. Stir in garlic and pepper flakes and cook until fragrant, about 30 seconds. Stir in wine, scraping up any browned bits, then stir in broth and pasta.
3. Lock lid in place and close pressure release valve. Select high pressure cook function and cook for 4 minutes. Turn off Instant Pot and quick-release pressure. Carefully remove lid, allowing steam to escape away from you.
4. Stir broccoli rabe and any accumulated juices and Parmesan into pasta. Season with salt and pepper to taste. Serve, passing extra Parmesan separately.

Per Serving
calories: 440 | fat: 12g | protein: 22g
carbs: 59g | fiber: 1g | sodium: 930mg

Orzo with Shrimp and Feta Cheese

Prep time: 15 minutes | Cook time: 13 minutes | Serves 4 to 6

1 pound (454 g) large shrimp, peeled and deveined
1 tablespoon grated lemon zest plus 1 tablespoon juice
¼ teaspoon table salt
¼ teaspoon pepper
2 tablespoons extra-virgin olive oil, plus extra for serving
1 onion, chopped fine
2 garlic cloves, minced
2 cups orzo
2 cups chicken broth, plus extra as needed
1¼ cups water
½ cup pitted kalamata olives, chopped coarse
1 ounce (28 g) feta cheese, crumbled, plus extra for serving
1 tablespoon chopped fresh dill

1. Toss shrimp with lemon zest, salt, and pepper in bowl; refrigerate until ready to use.
2. Using highest sauté function, heat oil in Instant Pot until shimmering. Add onion and cook until softened, about 5 minutes. Stir in garlic and cook until fragrant, about 30 seconds. Add orzo and cook, stirring frequently, until orzo is coated with oil and lightly browned, about 5 minutes. Stir in broth and water, scraping up any browned bits.
3. Lock lid in place and close pressure release valve. Select high pressure cook function and cook for 2 minutes. Turn off Instant Pot and quick-release pressure. Carefully remove lid, allowing steam to escape away from you.
4. Stir shrimp, olives, and feta into orzo. Cover and let sit until shrimp are opaque throughout, 5 to 7 minutes. Adjust consistency with extra hot broth as needed. Stir in dill and lemon juice, and season with salt and pepper to taste. Sprinkle individual portions with extra feta and drizzle with extra oil before serving.

Per Serving
calories: 320 | fat: 7g | protein: 18g
carbs: 46g | fiber: 2g | sodium: 670mg

Triple-Green Pasta with Parmesan
Prep time: 10 minutes | Cook time: 14 minutes | Serves 4

8 ounces (227 g) uncooked penne
1 tablespoon extra-virgin olive oil
2 garlic cloves, minced
¼ teaspoon crushed red pepper
2 cups chopped fresh flat-leaf (Italian) parsley, including stems
5 cups loosely packed baby spinach)
¼ teaspoon ground nutmeg
¼ teaspoon freshly ground black pepper
¼ teaspoon kosher or sea salt
$^1/_3$ cup Castelvetrano olives, pitted and sliced
$^1/_3$ cup grated Pecorino Romano or Parmesan cheese

1. In a large stockpot, cook the pasta according to the package directions, but boil 1 minute less than instructed. Drain the pasta, and save ¼ cup of the cooking water.
2. While the pasta is cooking, in a large skillet over medium heat, heat the oil. Add the garlic and crushed red pepper, and cook for 30 seconds, stirring constantly. Add the parsley and cook for 1 minute, stirring constantly. Add the spinach, nutmeg, pepper, and salt, and cook for 3 minutes, stirring occasionally, until the spinach is wilted.
3. Add the pasta and the reserved ¼ cup pasta water to the skillet. Stir in the olives, and cook for about 2 minutes, until most of the pasta water has been absorbed. Remove from the heat, stir in the cheese, and serve.

Per Serving
calories: 262 | fat: 3g | protein: 15g
carbs: 51g | fiber: 12g | sodium: 1180mg

Asparagus and Grape Tomato Pasta
Prep time: 10 minutes | Cook time: 25 minutes | Serves 6

8 ounces (227 g) uncooked small pasta, like orecchiette (little ears) or farfalle (bow ties)
1½ pounds (680 g) fresh asparagus, ends trimmed and stalks chopped into 1-inch pieces
1½ cups grape tomatoes, halved
2 tablespoons extra-virgin olive oil
¼ teaspoon freshly ground black pepper
¼ teaspoon kosher or sea salt
2 cups fresh Mozzarella, drained and cut into bite-size pieces
$^1/_3$ cup torn fresh basil leaves
2 tablespoons balsamic vinegar

1. Preheat the oven to 400ºF (205ºC).
2. In a large stockpot, cook the pasta according to the package directions. Drain, reserving about ¼ cup of the pasta water.
3. While the pasta is cooking, in a large bowl, toss the asparagus, tomatoes, oil, pepper, and salt together. Spread the mixture onto a large, rimmed baking sheet and bake for 15 minutes, stirring twice as it cooks.
4. Remove the vegetables from the oven, and add the cooked pasta to the baking sheet. Mix with a few tablespoons of pasta water to help the sauce become smoother and the saucy vegetables stick to the pasta.
5. Gently mix in the Mozzarella and basil. Drizzle with the balsamic vinegar. Serve from the baking sheet or pour the pasta into a large bowl.
6. If you want to make this dish ahead of time or to serve it cold, follow the recipe up to step 4, then refrigerate the pasta and vegetables. When you are ready to serve, follow step 5 either with the cold pasta or with warm pasta that's been gently reheated in a pot on the stove.

Per Serving
calories: 147 | fat: 2g | protein: 16g
carbs: 17g | fiber: 4g | sodium: 420mg

Creamy Garlic Parmesan Chicken Pasta

Prep time: 5 minutes | Cook time: 15 minutes | Serves 4

3 tablespoons extra-virgin olive oil
2 boneless, skinless chicken breasts, cut into thin strips
1 large onion, thinly sliced
3 tablespoons garlic, minced
1½ teaspoons salt
1 pound (454 g) fettuccine pasta
1 cup heavy whipping cream
¾ cup freshly grated Parmesan cheese, divided
½ teaspoon freshly ground black pepper

1. In a large skillet over medium heat, heat the olive oil. Add the chicken and cook for 3 minutes.
2. Add the onion, garlic and salt to the skillet. Cook for 7 minutes, stirring occasionally.
3. Meanwhile, bring a large pot of salted water to a boil and add the pasta, then cook for 7 minutes.
4. While the pasta is cooking, add the heavy cream, ½ cup of the Parmesan cheese and black pepper to the chicken. Simmer for 3 minutes.
5. Reserve ½ cup of the pasta water. Drain the pasta and add it to the chicken cream sauce.
6. Add the reserved pasta water to the pasta and toss together. Simmer for 2 minutes. Top with the remaining ¼ cup of the Parmesan cheese and serve warm.

Per Serving
calories: 879 | fat: 42g | protein: 35g
carbs: 90g | fiber: 5g | sodium: 1283mg

Dinner Meaty Baked Penne

Prep time: 5 minutes | Cook time: 50 minutes | Serves 8

1 pound (454 g) penne pasta
1 pound (454 g) ground beef
1 teaspoon salt
1 (25-ounce / 709-g) jar marinara sauce
1 (1-pound / 454-g) bag baby spinach, washed
3 cups shredded Mozzarella cheese, divided

1. Bring a large pot of salted water to a boil, add the penne, and cook for 7 minutes. Reserve 2 cups of the pasta water and drain the pasta.
2. Preheat the oven to 350ºF (180ºC).
3. In a large saucepan over medium heat, cook the ground beef and salt. Brown the ground beef for about 5 minutes.
4. Stir in marinara sauce, and 2 cups of pasta water. Let simmer for 5 minutes.
5. Add a handful of spinach at a time into the sauce, and cook for another 3 minutes.
6. To assemble, in a 9-by-13-inch baking dish, add the pasta and pour the pasta sauce over it. Stir in 1½ cups of the Mozzarella cheese. Cover the dish with foil and bake for 20 minutes.
7. After 20 minutes, remove the foil, top with the rest of the Mozzarella, and bake for another 10 minutes. Serve warm.

Per Serving
calories: 497 | fat: 17g | protein: 31g
carbs: 54g | fiber: 4g | sodium: 619mg

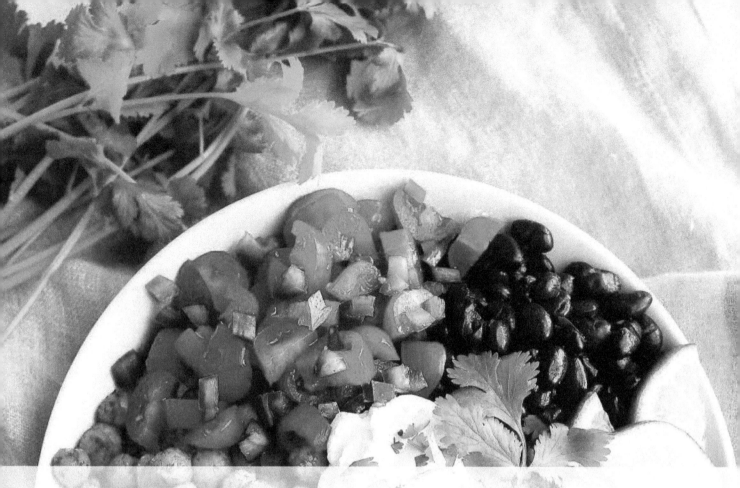
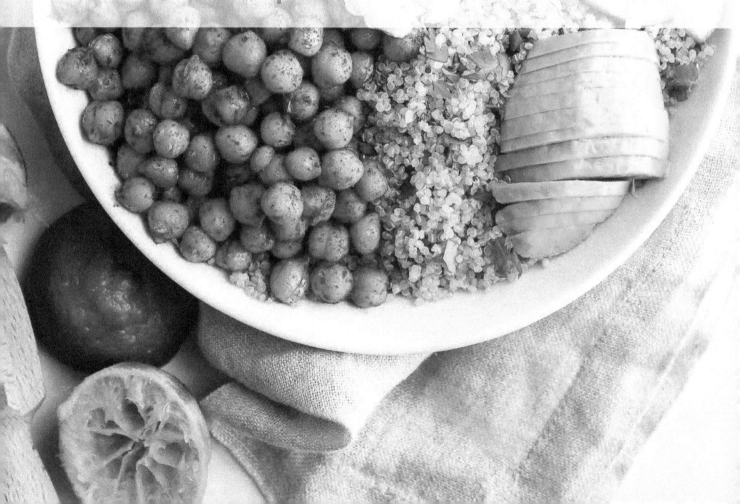

Chapter 15 Salads

Tomato and Lentil Salad with Feta

Prep time: 10 minutes | Cook time: 30 minutes | Serves 4

3 cups water
1 cup brown or green lentils, picked over and rinsed
1½ teaspoons salt, divided
2 large ripe tomatoes

2 Persian cucumbers
1/3 cup lemon juice
½ cup extra-virgin olive oil
1 cup crumbled feta cheese

1. In a large pot over medium heat, bring the water, lentils, and 1 teaspoon of salt to a simmer, then reduce heat to low. Cover the pot and continue to cook, stirring occasionally, for 30 minutes. (The lentils should be cooked so that they no longer have a crunch, but still hold their form. You should be able to smooth the lentil between your two fingers when pinched.)
2. Once the lentils are done cooking, strain them to remove any excess water and put them into a large bowl. Let cool.
3. Dice the tomatoes and cucumbers, then add them to the lentils.
4. In a small bowl, whisk together the lemon juice, olive oil, and remaining ½ teaspoon salt.
5. Pour the dressing over the lentils and vegetables. Add the feta cheese to the bowl, and gently toss all of the ingredients together.

Per Serving
calories: 521 | fat: 36g | protein: 18g
carbs: 35g | fiber: 15g | sodium: 1304mg

Quinoa and Garbanzo Salad

Prep time: 10 minutes | Cook time: 30 minutes | Serves 8

4 cups water
2 cups red or yellow quinoa
2 teaspoons salt, divided
1 cup thinly sliced onions (red or white)
1 (16-ounce / 454-g)

can garbanzo beans, rinsed and drained
1/3 cup extra-virgin olive oil
¼ cup lemon juice
1 teaspoon freshly ground black pepper

1. In a 3-quart pot over medium heat, bring the water to a boil.
2. Add the quinoa and 1 teaspoon of salt to the pot. Stir, cover, and let cook over low heat for 15 to 20 minutes.
3. Turn off the heat, fluff the quinoa with a fork, cover again, and let stand for 5 to 10 more minutes.
4. Put the cooked quinoa, onions, and garbanzo beans in a large bowl.
5. In a separate small bowl, whisk together the olive oil, lemon juice, remaining 1 teaspoon of salt, and black pepper.
6. Add the dressing to the quinoa mixture and gently toss everything together. Serve warm or cold.

Per Serving
calories: 318 | fat: 6g | protein: 9g
carbs: 43g | fiber: 13g | sodium: 585mg

Zesty Spanish Potato Salad

Prep time: 10 minutes | Cook time: 5 to 7 minutes | Serves 6 to 8

4 russet potatoes, peeled and chopped
3 large hard-boiled eggs, chopped
1 cup frozen mixed vegetables, thawed
½ cup plain, unsweetened, full-fat Greek yogurt
5 tablespoons pitted

Spanish olives
½ teaspoon freshly ground black pepper
½ teaspoon dried mustard seed
½ tablespoon freshly squeezed lemon juice
½ teaspoon dried dill
Salt, to taste

1. Place the potatoes in a large pot of water and boil for 5 to 7 minutes, until just fork-tender, checking periodically for doneness. You don't have to overcook them.
2. Meanwhile, in a large bowl, mix the eggs, vegetables, yogurt, olives, pepper, mustard, lemon juice, and dill. Season with salt to taste. Once the potatoes are cooled somewhat, add them to the large bowl, then toss well and serve.

Per Serving
calories: 192 | fat: 5g | protein: 9g
carbs: 30g | fiber: 2g | sodium: 59mg

Winter Salad with Red Wine Vinaigrette

Prep time: 10 minutes | Cook time: 0 minutes | Serves 4

1 small green apple, thinly sliced
6 stalks kale, stems removed and greens roughly chopped
½ cup crumbled feta cheese
½ cup dried currants
½ cup chopped pitted Kalamata olives
½ cup thinly sliced radicchio
2 scallions, both green and white parts, thinly sliced
¼ cup peeled, julienned carrots
2 celery stalks, thinly sliced
¼ cup Red Wine Vinaigrette
Salt and freshly ground black pepper, to taste (optional)

1. In a large bowl, combine the apple, kale, feta, currants, olives, radicchio, scallions, carrots, and celery and mix well. Drizzle with the vinaigrette. Season with salt and pepper (if using), then serve.

Per Serving
calories: 253 | fat: 15g | protein: 6g
carbs: 29g | fiber: 4g | sodium: 480mg

Avocado and Hearts of Palm Salad

Prep time: 10 minutes | Cook time: 0 minutes | Serves 4

2 (14-ounce / 397-g) cans hearts of palm, drained and cut into ½-inch-thick slices
1 avocado, cut into ½-inch pieces
1 cup halved yellow cherry tomatoes
½ small shallot, thinly sliced
¼ cup coarsely chopped flat-leaf parsley
2 tablespoons low-fat mayonnaise
2 tablespoons extra-virgin olive oil
¼ teaspoon salt
⅛ teaspoon freshly ground black pepper

1. In a large bowl, toss the hearts of palm, avocado, tomatoes, shallot, and parsley.
2. In a small bowl, whisk the mayonnaise, olive oil, salt, and pepper, then mix into the large bowl.

Per Serving
calories: 192 | fat: 15g | protein: 5g
carbs: 14g | fiber: 7g | sodium: 841mg

Arugula, Watermelon, and Feta Salad

Prep time: 10 minutes | Cook time: 0 minutes | Serves 2

3 cups packed arugula
2½ cups watermelon, cut into bite-size cubes
2 ounces (57 g) feta cheese, crumbled
2 tablespoons balsamic glaze

1. Divide the arugula between two plates.
2. Divide the watermelon cubes between the beds of arugula.
3. Sprinkle 1 ounce (28 g) of the feta over each salad.
4. Drizzle about 1 tablespoon of the glaze (or more if desired) over each salad.

Per Serving
calories: 159 | fat: 7g | protein: 6g
carbs: 21g | fiber: 1g | sodium: 327mg

Greek Vegetable Salad

Prep time: 10 minutes | Cook time: 0 minutes | Serves 4 to 6

1 head iceberg lettuce
2 cups cherry tomatoes
1 large cucumber
1 medium onion
½ cup extra-virgin olive oil
¼ cup lemon juice
1 teaspoon salt
1 clove garlic, minced
1 cup Kalamata olives, pitted
1 (6-ounce / 170-g) package feta cheese, crumbled

1. Cut the lettuce into 1-inch pieces and put them in a large salad bowl.
2. Cut the tomatoes in half and add them to the salad bowl.
3. Slice the cucumber into bite-size pieces and add them to the salad bowl.
4. Thinly slice the onion and add it to the salad bowl.
5. In another small bowl, whisk together the olive oil, lemon juice, salt, and garlic. Pour the dressing over the salad and gently toss to evenly coat.
6. Top the salad with the Kalamata olives and feta cheese and serve.

Per Serving
calories: 539 | fat: 50g | protein: 9g
carbs: 17g | fiber: 4g | sodium: 1758mg

Tuna Salad

Prep time: 10 minutes | Cook time: 0 minutes | Serves 4

4 cups spring mix greens
1 (15-ounce / 425-g) can cannellini beans, drained
2 (5-ounce / 142-g) cans water-packed, white albacore tuna, drained
²⁄₃ cup crumbled feta cheese
½ cup thinly sliced sun-dried tomatoes
¼ cup sliced pitted Kalamata olives

¼ cup thinly sliced scallions, both green and white parts
3 tablespoons extra-virgin olive oil
½ teaspoon dried cilantro
2 or 3 leaves thinly chopped fresh sweet basil
1 lime, zested and juiced
Kosher salt and freshly ground black pepper, to taste

1. In a large bowl, combine greens, beans, tuna, feta, tomatoes, olives, scallions, olive oil, cilantro, basil, and lime juice and zest. Season with salt and pepper, mix, and enjoy!

Per Serving (1 cup)
calories: 355 | fat: 19g | protein: 22g
carbs: 25g | fiber: 8g | sodium: 744mg

Balsamic Baby Spinach Salad

Prep time: 10 minutes | Cook time: 0 minutes | Serves 4

1 large ripe tomato
1 medium red onion
½ teaspoon fresh lemon zest
3 tablespoons balsamic vinegar

¼ cup extra-virgin olive oil
½ teaspoon salt
1 pound (454 g) baby spinach, washed, stems removed

1. Dice the tomato into ¼-inch pieces and slice the onion into long slivers.
2. In a small bowl, whisk together the lemon zest, balsamic vinegar, olive oil, and salt.
3. Put the spinach, tomatoes, and onions in a large bowl. Pour the dressing over the salad and lightly toss to coat.

Per Serving
calories: 172 | fat: 14g | protein: 4g
carbs: 9g | fiber: 4g | sodium: 389mg

Orange Avocado and Almond Salad

Prep time: 10 minutes | Cook time: 0 minutes | Serves 5 to 6

2 large Gala apples, chopped
2 oranges, segmented and chopped
¹⁄₃ cup sliced almonds
½ cup honey

1 tablespoon extra-virgin olive oil
½ teaspoon grated orange zest
1 large avocado, semi-ripened, medium diced

1. In a large bowl, combine the apples, oranges, and almonds. Mix gently.
2. In a small bowl, whisk the honey, oil, and orange zest. Set aside.
3. Drizzle the orange zest mix over the fruit salad and toss. Add the avocado and toss gently one more time.

Per Serving
calories: 296 | fat: 12g | protein: 3g
carbs: 50g | fiber: 7g | sodium: 4mg

Arugula and Walnut Salad

Prep time: 10 minutes | Cook time: 0 minutes | Serves 4

4 tablespoons extra-virgin olive oil
Zest and juice of 2 clementines or 1 orange (2 to 3 tablespoons)
1 tablespoon red wine vinegar
½ teaspoon salt

¼ teaspoon freshly ground black pepper
8 cups baby arugula
1 cup coarsely chopped walnuts
1 cup crumbled goat cheese
½ cup pomegranate seeds

1. In a small bowl, whisk together the olive oil, zest and juice, vinegar, salt, and pepper and set aside.
2. To assemble the salad for serving, in a large bowl, combine the arugula, walnuts, goat cheese, and pomegranate seeds. Drizzle with the dressing and toss to coat.

Per Serving
calories: 444 | fat: 40g | protein: 10g
carbs: 11g | fiber: 3g | sodium: 412mg

Kale Salad with Anchovy Dressing

Prep time: 15 minutes | Cook time: 0 minutes | Serves 4

1 large bunch lacinato or dinosaur kale
¼ cup toasted pine nuts
1 cup shaved or coarsely shredded fresh Parmesan cheese
¼ cup extra-virgin

olive oil
8 anchovy fillets, roughly chopped
2 to 3 tablespoons freshly squeezed lemon juice (from 1 large lemon)
2 teaspoons red pepper flakes (optional)

1. Remove the rough center stems from the kale leaves and roughly tear each leaf into about 4-by-1-inch strips. Place the torn kale in a large bowl and add the pine nuts and cheese.
2. In a small bowl, whisk together the olive oil, anchovies, lemon juice, and red pepper flakes (if using). Drizzle over the salad and toss to coat well. Let sit at room temperature 30 minutes before serving, tossing again just prior to serving.

Per Serving
calories: 337 | fat: 25g | protein: 16g
carbs: 12g | fiber: 2g | sodium: 603mg

Authentic Greek Salad

Prep time: 10 minutes | Cook time: 0 minutes | Serves 4

2 large English cucumbers
4 Roma tomatoes, quartered
1 green bell pepper, cut into 1- to 1½-inch chunks
¼ small red onion, thinly sliced
4 ounces (113 g) pitted Kalamata olives
¼ cup extra-virgin olive oil

2 tablespoons freshly squeezed lemon juice
1 tablespoon red wine vinegar
1 tablespoon chopped fresh oregano or 1 teaspoon dried oregano
¼ teaspoon freshly ground black pepper
4 ounces (113 g) crumbled traditional feta cheese

1. Cut the cucumbers in half lengthwise and then into ½-inch-thick half-moons. Place in a large bowl.
2. Add the quartered tomatoes, bell pepper, red onion, and olives.
3. In a small bowl, whisk together the olive oil, lemon juice, vinegar, oregano, and pepper. Drizzle over the vegetables and toss to coat.
4. Divide between salad plates and top each with 1 ounce (28 g) of feta.

Per Serving
calories: 278 | fat: 22g | protein: 8g
carbs: 12g | fiber: 4g | sodium: 572mg

Citrus Fennel and Pecan Salad

Prep time: 10 minutes | Cook time: 0 minutes | Serves 2

For the Dressing:
2 tablespoons fresh orange juice
3 tablespoons olive oil
1 tablespoon blood orange vinegar, other

orange vinegar, or cider vinegar
1 tablespoon honey
Salt, to taste
Freshly ground black pepper, to taste

For the Salad:
2 cups packed baby kale
1 medium navel or blood orange, segmented
½ small fennel bulb, stems and leaves

removed, sliced into matchsticks
3 tablespoons toasted pecans, chopped
2 ounces (57 g) goat cheese, crumbled

Make the Dressing
1. Combine the orange juice, olive oil, vinegar, and honey in a small bowl and whisk to combine. Season with salt and pepper. Set the dressing aside.

Make the Salad
2. Divide the baby kale, orange segments, fennel, pecans, and goat cheese evenly between two plates.
3. Drizzle half of the dressing over each salad.

Per Serving
calories: 502 | fat: 39g | protein: 13g
carbs: 30g | fiber: 6g | sodium: 158mg

Tabouli Salad

Prep time: 10 minutes | Cook time: 0 minutes | Serves 8 to 10

1 cup bulgur wheat, grind
4 cups Italian parsley, finely chopped
2 cups ripe tomato, finely diced
1 cup green onion, finely chopped
½ cup lemon juice
½ cup extra-virgin olive oil
1½ teaspoons salt
1 teaspoon dried mint

1. Before you chop the vegetables, put the bulgur in a small bowl. Rinse with water, drain, and let stand in the bowl while you prepare the other ingredients.
2. Put the parsley, tomatoes, green onion, and bulgur into a large bowl.
3. In a small bowl, whisk together the lemon juice, olive oil, salt, and mint.
4. Pour the dressing over the tomato, onion, and bulgur mixture, tossing everything together. Add additional salt to taste. Serve immediately or store in the fridge for up to 2 days.

Per Serving
calories: 207 | fat: 14g | protein: 4g
carbs: 19g | fiber: 5g | sodium: 462mg

Panzanella Salad

Prep time: 10 minutes | Cook time: 11 minutes | Serves 2

Cooking spray
1 ear corn on the cob, peeled and shucked
4 slices stale French baguette
½ pint cherry or grape tomatoes, halved
1 medium sweet pepper, seeded and cut into 1-inch pieces
1 medium avocado, pitted and cut into
cubes
4 very thin slices of sweet onion, cut crosswise into thin rings
½ cup fresh whole basil leaves
2 ounces (57 g) mini Mozzarella balls (ciliegine), halved or quartered
¼ cup honey balsamic dressing

1. Heat the grill to medium-high heat (about 350ºF (180ºC)) and lightly spray the cooking grates with cooking spray.

2. Grill the corn for 10 minutes, or until it is lightly charred all around.
3. Grill the bread for 30 to 45 seconds on each side, or until it has grill marks.
4. Let the corn sit until it's cool enough to handle. Cut the kernels off the cob and place them in a large bowl.
5. Cut the bread into chunks and add it to the bowl.
6. Add the tomatoes, sweet pepper, avocado, onion, basil, Mozzarella, and dressing to the bowl, and toss lightly to combine. Let the salad sit for about 15 minutes in the refrigerator, so the bread can soften and the flavors can blend.
7. This is best served shortly after it's prepared.

Per Serving
calories: 525 | fat: 26g | protein: 16g
carbs: 60g | fiber: 10g | sodium: 524mg

Fig, Prosciutto and Arugula Salad

Prep time: 10 minutes | Cook time: 1 minute | Serves 2

3 cups arugula
4 fresh, ripe figs (or 4 to 6 dried figs), stemmed and sliced
2 tablespoons olive oil
3 very thin slices prosciutto, trimmed of any fat and sliced
lengthwise into 1-inch strips
¼ cup pecan halves, lightly toasted
2 tablespoons crumbled blue cheese
1 to 2 tablespoons balsamic glaze

1. In a large bowl, toss the arugula and figs with the olive oil.
2. Place the prosciutto on a microwave-safe plate and heat it on high in the microwave for 60 seconds, or until it just starts to crisp.
3. Add the crisped prosciutto, pecans, and blue cheese to the bowl. Toss the salad lightly.
4. Drizzle with the balsamic glaze.

Per Serving
calories: 519 | fat: 38g | protein: 20g
carbs: 29g | fiber: 6g | sodium: 482mg

Pistachio-Parmesan Kale and Arugula Salad

Prep time: 10 minutes | Cook time: minutes | Serves 6

6 cups raw kale, center ribs removed and discarded, leaves coarsely chopped
¼ cup extra-virgin olive oil
2 tablespoons freshly squeezed lemon juice
½ teaspoon smoked paprika
2 cups arugula
⅓ cup unsalted shelled pistachios
6 tablespoons grated Parmesan or Pecorino Romano cheese

1. In a large salad bowl, combine the kale, oil, lemon juice, and smoked paprika. With your hands, gently massage the leaves for about 15 seconds or so, until all are thoroughly coated. Let the kale sit for 10 minutes.
2. When you're ready to serve, gently mix in the arugula and pistachios. Divide the salad among six serving bowls, sprinkle 1 tablespoon of grated cheese over each, and serve.

Per Serving
calories: 105 | fat: 9g | protein: 4g
carbs: 3g | fiber: 2g | sodium: 176mg

Tricolor Summer Salad

Prep time: 10 minutes | Cook time: 0 minutes | Serves 3 to 4

¼ cup while balsamic vinegar
2 tablespoons Dijon mustard
1 tablespoon sugar
½ teaspoon garlic salt
½ teaspoon freshly ground black pepper
¼ cup extra-virgin
olive oil
1½ cups chopped orange, yellow, and red tomatoes
½ cucumber, peeled and diced
1 small red onion, thinly sliced
¼ cup crumbled feta (optional)

1. In a small bowl, whisk the vinegar, mustard, sugar, pepper, and garlic salt. Then slowly whisk in the olive oil.
2. In a large bowl, add the tomatoes, cucumber, and red onion. Add the dressing. Toss once or twice, and serve with the feta crumbles (if desired) sprinkled on top.

Per Serving
calories: 246 | fat: 18g | protein: 1g
carbs: 19g | fiber: 2g | sodium: 483mg

Cauliflower Tabbouleh Salad

Prep time: 15 minutes | Cook time: 5 minutes | Serves 6

6 tablespoons extra-virgin olive oil, divided
4 cups riced cauliflower
3 garlic cloves, finely minced
1½ teaspoons salt
½ teaspoon freshly ground black pepper
½ large cucumber, peeled, seeded, and chopped
½ cup chopped mint leaves
½ cup chopped
Italian parsley
½ cup chopped pitted Kalamata olives
2 tablespoons minced red onion
Juice of 1 lemon (about 2 tablespoons)
2 cups baby arugula or spinach leaves
2 medium avocados, peeled, pitted, and diced
1 cup quartered cherry tomatoes

1. In a large skillet, heat 2 tablespoons of olive oil over medium-high heat. Add the riced cauliflower, garlic, salt, and pepper and sauté until just tender but not mushy, 3 to 4 minutes. Remove from the heat and place in a large bowl.
2. Add the cucumber, mint, parsley, olives, red onion, lemon juice, and remaining 4 tablespoons olive oil and toss well. Place in the refrigerator, uncovered, and refrigerate for at least 30 minutes, or up to 2 hours.
3. Before serving, add the arugula, avocado, and tomatoes and toss to combine well. Season to taste with salt and pepper and serve cold or at room temperature.

Per Serving
calories: 235 | fat: 21g | protein: 4g
carbs: 12g | fiber: 6g | sodium: 623mg

Italian Celery and Orange Salad

Prep time: 10 minutes | Cook time: 0 minutes | Serves 6

3 celery stalks, including leaves, sliced diagonally into ½-inch slices
2 large oranges, peeled and sliced into rounds
½ cup green olives (or any variety)
¼ cup sliced red onion
1 tablespoon extra-virgin olive oil
1 tablespoon olive brine
1 tablespoon freshly squeezed lemon or orange juice
¼ teaspoon kosher or sea salt
¼ teaspoon freshly ground black pepper

1. Place the celery, oranges, olives, and onion on a large serving platter or in a shallow, wide bowl.
2. In a small bowl, whisk together the oil, olive brine, and lemon juice. Pour over the salad, sprinkle with salt and pepper, and serve.

Per Serving
calories: 21 | fat: 1g | protein: 1g
carbs: 1g | fiber: 1g | sodium: 138mg

Cantaloupe Caprese Salad

Prep time: 10 minutes | Cook time: 0 minutes | Serves 6

1 cantaloupe, quartered and seeded
½ small seedless watermelon
1 cup grape tomatoes
2 cups fresh Mozzarella balls
⅓ cup fresh basil or mint leaves, torn into
small pieces
2 tablespoons extra-virgin olive oil
1 tablespoon balsamic vinegar
¼ teaspoon freshly ground black pepper
¼ teaspoon kosher or sea salt

1. Using a melon baller or a metal, teaspoon-size measuring spoon, scoop balls out of the cantaloupe. You should get about 2½ to 3 cups from one cantaloupe. (If you prefer, cut the melon into bite-size pieces instead of making balls.) Put them in a large colander over a large serving bowl.
2. Using the same method, ball or cut the watermelon into bite-size pieces; you should get about 2 cups. Put the watermelon balls in the colander with the cantaloupe.

3. Let the fruit drain for 10 minutes. Pour the juice from the bowl into a container to refrigerate and save for drinking or adding to smoothies. Wipe the bowl dry, and put in the cut fruit.
4. Add the tomatoes, Mozzarella, basil, oil, vinegar, pepper, and salt to the fruit mixture. Gently mix until everything is incorporated and serve.

Per Serving
calories: 58 | fat: 2g | protein: 1g
carbs: 8g | fiber: 1g | sodium: 156mg

Israeli Salad

Prep time: 15 minutes | Cook time: 6 minutes | Serves 4

¼ cup pine nuts
¼ cup shelled pistachios
¼ cup coarsely chopped walnuts
¼ cup shelled pumpkin seeds
¼ cup shelled sunflower seeds
2 large English cucumbers, unpeeled and finely chopped
1 pint cherry tomatoes, finely chopped
½ small red onion, finely chopped
½ cup finely chopped fresh flat-leaf Italian parsley
¼ cup extra-virgin olive oil
2 to 3 tablespoons freshly squeezed lemon juice (from 1 lemon)
1 teaspoon salt
¼ teaspoon freshly ground black pepper
4 cups baby arugula

1. In a large dry skillet, toast the pine nuts, pistachios, walnuts, pumpkin seeds, and sunflower seeds over medium-low heat until golden and fragrant, 5 to 6 minutes, being careful not to burn them. Remove from the heat and set aside.
2. In a large bowl, combine the cucumber, tomatoes, red onion, and parsley.
3. In a small bowl, whisk together olive oil, lemon juice, salt, and pepper. Pour over the chopped vegetables and toss to coat.
4. Add the toasted nuts and seeds and arugula and toss with the salad to blend well. Serve at room temperature or chilled.

Per Serving
calories: 414 | fat: 34g | protein: 10g
carbs: 17g | fiber: 6g | sodium: 642mg

Beet Summer Salad

Prep time: 20 minutes | Cook time: 40 minutes | Serves 4 to 6

6 medium to large fresh red or yellow beets
1/3 cup plus 1 tablespoon extra-virgin olive oil, divided
4 heads of Treviso
radicchio
2 shallots, peeled and sliced
1/4 cup lemon juice
1/2 teaspoon salt
6 ounces (170 g) feta cheese, crumbled

1. Preheat the oven to 400°F (205°C).
2. Cut off the stems and roots of the beets. Wash the beets thoroughly and dry them off with a paper towel.
3. Peel the beets using a vegetable peeler. Cut into 1/2-inch pieces and put them into a large bowl.
4. Add 1 tablespoon of olive oil to the bowl and toss to coat, then pour the beets out onto a baking sheet. Spread the beets so that they are evenly distributed.
5. Bake for 35 to 40 minutes until the beets are tender, turning once or twice with a spatula.
6. When the beets are done cooking, set them aside and let cool for 10 minutes.
7. While the beets are cooling, cut the radicchio into 1-inch pieces and place on a serving dish.
8. Once the beets have cooled, spoon them over the radicchio, then evenly distribute the shallots over the beets.
9. In a small bowl, whisk together the remaining 1/3 cup of olive oil, lemon juice, and salt. Drizzle the layered salad with dressing. Finish off the salad with feta cheese on top.

Per Serving
calories: 389 | fat: 31g | protein: 10g
carbs: 22g | fiber: 5g | sodium: 893mg

Tahini Barley Salad

Prep time: 20 minutes | Cook time: 8 minutes | Serves 4 to 6

1½ cups pearl barley
5 tablespoons extra-virgin olive oil, divided
1½ teaspoons table salt, for cooking barley
¼ cup tahini
1 teaspoon grated lemon zest plus ¼ cup juice (2 lemons)
1 tablespoon sumac, divided
1 garlic clove, minced
¾ teaspoon table salt
1 English cucumber, cut into ½-inch pieces
1 carrot, peeled and shredded
1 red bell pepper, stemmed, seeded, and chopped
4 scallions, thinly sliced
2 tablespoons finely chopped jarred hot cherry peppers
¼ cup coarsely chopped fresh mint

1. Combine 6 cups water, barley, 1 tablespoon oil, and 1½ teaspoons salt in Instant Pot. Lock lid in place and close pressure release valve. Select high pressure cook function and cook for 8 minutes. Turn off Instant Pot and let pressure release naturally for 15 minutes. Quick-release any remaining pressure, then carefully remove lid, allowing steam to escape away from you. Drain barley, spread onto rimmed baking sheet, and let cool completely, about 15 minutes.
2. Meanwhile, whisk remaining ¼ cup oil, tahini, 2 tablespoons water, lemon zest and juice, 1 teaspoon sumac, garlic, and ¾ teaspoon salt in large bowl until combined; let sit for 15 minutes.
3. Measure out and reserve ½ cup dressing for serving. Add barley, cucumber, carrot, bell pepper, scallions, and cherry peppers to bowl with dressing and gently toss to combine. Season with salt and pepper to taste. Transfer salad to serving dish and sprinkle with mint and remaining 2 teaspoons sumac. Serve, passing reserved dressing separately.

Per Serving
calories: 370 | fat: 18g | protein: 8g
carbs: 47g | fiber: 10g | sodium: 510mg

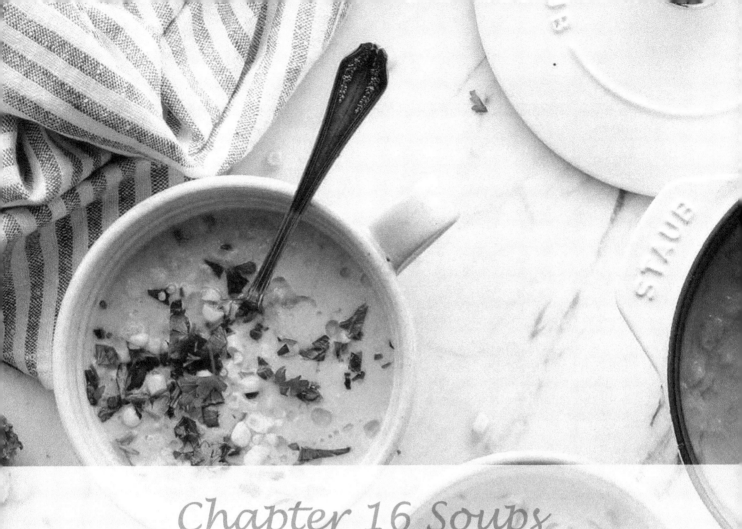

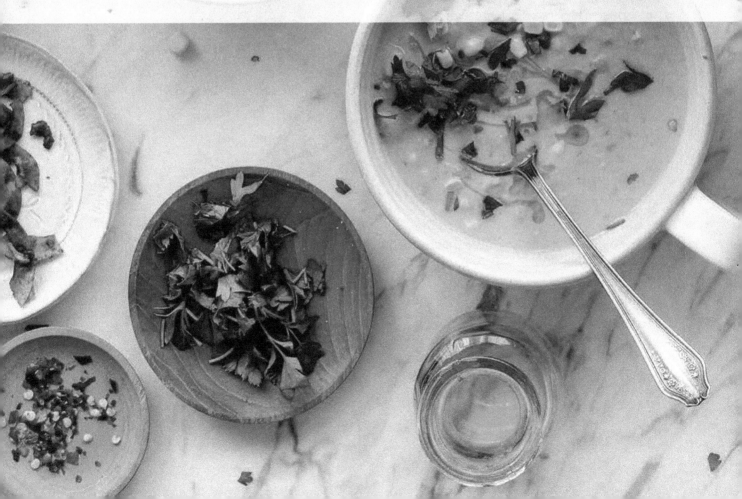

Chapter 16 Soups

Lemon Chicken Orzo Soup

Prep time: 10 minutes | Cook time: 20 minutes | Serves 8

1 tablespoon extra-virgin olive oil
1 cup chopped onion
½ cup chopped carrots
½ cup chopped celery
3 garlic cloves, minced
9 cups low-sodium chicken broth

2 cups shredded cooked chicken breast
½ cup freshly squeezed lemon juice
Zest of 1 lemon, grated
1 to 2 teaspoons dried oregano
8 ounces (227 g) cooked orzo pasta

1. In a large pot, heat the oil over medium heat and add the onion, carrots, celery, and garlic and cook for about 5 minutes, until the onions are translucent. Add the broth and bring to a boil.
2. Reduce to a simmer, cover, and cook for 10 more minutes, until the flavors meld. Then add the shredded chicken, lemon juice and zest, and oregano.
3. Plate the orzo in serving bowls first, then add the chicken soup.

Per Serving
calories: 215 | fat: 5g | protein: 16g
carbs: 27g | fiber: 2g | sodium: 114mg

Vegetable Gazpacho Soup

Prep time: 10 minutes | Cook time: 0 minutes | Serves 6 to 8

½ cup water
2 slices white bread, crust removed
2 pounds (907 g) ripe tomatoes
1 Persian cucumber, peeled and chopped
1 clove garlic, finely chopped

⅓ cup extra-virgin olive oil, plus more for garnish
2 tablespoons red wine vinegar
1 teaspoon salt
½ teaspoon freshly ground black pepper

1. Soak the bread in the water for 5 minutes; discard water when done.
2. Blend the bread, tomatoes, cucumber, garlic, olive oil, vinegar, salt, and black pepper in a food processor or blender until completely smooth.

3. Pour the soup into a glass container and store in the fridge until completely chilled.
4. When you are ready to serve, pour the soup into a bowl and top with a drizzle of olive oil.

Per Serving
calories: 163 | fat: 13g | protein: 2g
carbs: 12g | fiber: 2g | sodium: 442mg

Lentil Soup

Prep time: 25 minutes | Cook time: 1 hour 20 minutes | Serves 6 to 8

10 cups water
2 cups brown lentils, picked over and rinsed
2 teaspoons salt, divided
¼ cup long-grain rice, rinsed
3 tablespoons extra-

virgin olive oil
1 large onion, chopped
2 medium potatoes, peeled
1 teaspoon ground cumin
½ teaspoon freshly ground black pepper

1. In a large pot over medium heat, bring the water, lentils, and 1 teaspoon of salt to a simmer and continue to cook, stirring occasionally, for 30 minutes.
2. At the 30-minute mark, add the rice to the lentils. Cover and continue to simmer, stirring occasionally, for another 30 minutes.
3. Remove the pot from the heat and, using a handheld immersion blender, blend the lentils and rice for 1 to 2 minutes until smooth.
4. Return the pot to the stove over low heat.
5. In a small skillet over medium heat, cook the olive oil and onions for 5 minutes until the onions are golden brown. Add the onions to the soup.
6. Cut the potatoes into ¼-inch pieces and add them to the soup.
7. Add remaining 1 teaspoon of salt, cumin, and black pepper to the soup. Stir and continue to cook for 10 to 15 minutes, or until potatoes are thoroughly cooked. Serve warm.

Per Serving
calories: 348 | fat: 9g | protein: 18g
carbs: 53g | fiber: 20g | sodium: 795mg

Tomato Basil Soup

Prep time: 10 minutes | Cook time: 10 minutes | Serves 2

¼ cup extra-virgin olive oil
2 garlic cloves, minced
1 (14½-ounce / 411-g) can plum

tomatoes, whole or diced
1 cup vegetable broth
¼ cup chopped fresh basil

1. In a medium pot, heat the oil over medium heat, then add the garlic and cook for 2 minutes, until fragrant.
2. Meanwhile, in a bowl using an immersion blender or in a blender, purée the tomatoes and their juices.
3. Add the puréed tomatoes and broth to the pot and mix well. Simmer for 10 to 15 minutes and serve, garnished with basil.

Per Serving
calories: 307 | fat: 27g | protein: 3g
carbs: 11g | fiber: 4g | sodium: 661mg

White Bean Soup with Kale

Prep time: 25 minutes | Cook time: 30 minutes | Serves 4

1 to 2 tablespoons extra-virgin olive oil
1 large shallot, minced
1 large purple carrot, chopped
1 celery stalk, chopped
1 teaspoon garlic powder
3 cups low-sodium vegetable broth
1 (15-ounce / 425-g) can cannellini beans
1 cup chopped baby

kale
1 teaspoon salt (optional)
½ teaspoon freshly ground black pepper (optional)
1 lemon, juiced and zested
1½ tablespoons chopped fresh thyme (optional)
3 tablespoons chopped fresh oregano (optional)

1. In a large, deep pot, heat the oil. Add the shallot, carrot, celery, and garlic powder and sauté on medium-low heat for 3 to 5 minutes, until the vegetables are golden.
2. Add the vegetable broth and beans and bring to a simmer. Cook for 15 minutes.

3. Add in the kale, salt (if using), and pepper (if using). Cook for another 5 to 10 minutes, until the kale is soft. Right before serving, stir in the lemon juice and zest, thyme (if using), and oregano (if using).

Per Serving
calories: 165 | fat: 4g | protein: 7g
carbs: 26g | fiber: 7g | sodium: 135mg

Beans and Kale Fagioli

Prep time: 15 minutes | Cook time: 46 minutes | Serves 2

1 tablespoon olive oil
2 medium carrots, diced
2 medium celery stalks, diced
½ medium onion, diced
1 large garlic clove, minced
3 tablespoons tomato paste
4 cups low-sodium vegetable broth
1 cup packed kale,

stemmed and chopped
1 (15-ounce / 425-g) can red kidney beans, drained and rinsed
1 (15-ounce / 425-g) can cannellini beans, drained and rinsed
½ cup fresh basil, chopped
Salt, to taste
Freshly ground black pepper, to taste

1. Heat the olive oil in a stockpot over medium-high heat. Add the carrots, celery, onion, and garlic and sauté for 10 minutes, or until the vegetables start to turn golden.
2. Stir in the tomato paste and cook for about 30 seconds.
3. Add the vegetable broth and bring the soup to a boil. Cover, and reduce the heat to low. Cook the soup for 45 minutes, or until the carrots are tender.
4. Using an immersion blender, purée the soup so that it's partly smooth, but with some chunks of vegetables. If you don't have an immersion blender, scoop out about ⅓ of the soup and blend it in a blender, then add it back to the pot.
5. Add the kale, beans, and basil. Season with salt and pepper.

Per Serving
calories: 215 | fat: 4g | protein: 11g
carbs: 35g | fiber: 11g | sodium: 486mg

Greek Chicken Artichoke Soup

Prep time: 10 minutes | Cook time: 15 minutes | Serves 4

4 cups chicken stock
2 cups riced cauliflower, divided
2 large egg yolks
¼ cup freshly squeezed lemon juice (about 2 lemons)
¾ cup extra-virgin olive oil, divided
8 ounces (227 g) cooked chicken, coarsely chopped
1 (13¾-ounce / 390-g) can artichoke hearts, drained and quartered
¼ cup chopped fresh dill

1. In a large saucepan, bring the stock to a low boil. Reduce the heat to low and simmer, covered.
2. Transfer 1 cup of the hot stock to a blender or food processor. Add ½ cup raw riced cauliflower, the egg yolks, and lemon juice and purée. While the processor or blender is running, stream in ½ cup olive oil and blend until smooth.
3. Whisking constantly, pour the purée into the simmering stock until well blended together and smooth. Add the chicken and artichokes and simmer until thickened slightly, 8 to 10 minutes. Stir in the dill and remaining 1½ cups riced cauliflower. Serve warm, drizzled with the remaining ¼ cup olive oil.

Per Serving
calories: 566 | fat: 46g | protein: 24g
carbs: 14g | fiber: 7g | sodium: 754mg

Tomato Hummus Soup

Prep time: 10 minutes | Cook time: 10 minutes | Serves 2

1 (14½-ounce / 411-g) can crushed tomatoes with basil
1 cup roasted red pepper hummus
2 cups low-sodium chicken stock
Salt, to taste
¼ cup fresh basil leaves, thinly sliced (optional, for garnish)
Garlic croutons (optional, for garnish)

1. Combine the canned tomatoes, hummus, and chicken stock in a blender and blend until smooth. Pour the mixture into a saucepan and bring it to a boil.
2. Season with salt and fresh basil if desired. Serve with garlic croutons as a garnish, if desired.

Per Serving
calories: 148 | fat: 6g | protein: 5g
carbs: 19g | fiber: 4g | sodium: 680mg

Farro, Pancetta, and Leek Soup

Prep time: 10 minutes | Cook time: 16 minutes | Serves 6 to 8

1 cup whole farro
1 tablespoon extra-virgin olive oil, plus extra for drizzling
3 ounces (85 g) pancetta, chopped fine
1 pound (454 g) leeks, ends trimmed, chopped, and washed
thoroughly
2 carrots, peeled and chopped
1 celery rib, chopped
8 cups chicken broth, plus extra as needed
½ cup minced fresh parsley
Grated Parmesan cheese

1. Pulse farro in blender until about half of grains are broken into smaller pieces, about 6 pulses; set aside.
2. Using highest sauté function, heat oil in Instant Pot until shimmering. Add pancetta and cook until lightly browned, 3 to 5 minutes. Stir in leeks, carrots, and celery and cook until softened, about 5 minutes. Stir in broth, scraping up any browned bits, then stir in farro.
3. Lock lid in place and close pressure release valve. Select high pressure cook function and cook for 8 minutes. Turn off Instant Pot and quick-release pressure. Carefully remove lid, allowing steam to escape away from you.
4. Adjust consistency with extra hot broth as needed. Stir in parsley and season with salt and pepper to taste. Drizzle individual portions with extra oil and top with Parmesan before serving.

Per Serving
calories: 180 | fat: 6g | protein: 22g
carbs: 24g | fiber: 1g | sodium: 950mg

Avocado and Tomato Gazpacho

Prep time: 15 minutes | Cook time: 0 minutes | Serves 4

2 cups chopped tomatoes
2 large ripe avocados, halved and pitted
1 large cucumber, peeled and seeded
1 medium bell pepper (red, orange or yellow), chopped
1 cup plain whole-milk Greek yogurt
¼ cup extra-virgin olive oil
¼ cup chopped fresh cilantro
¼ cup chopped scallions, green part only
2 tablespoons red wine vinegar
Juice of 2 limes or 1 lemon
½ to 1 teaspoon salt
¼ teaspoon freshly ground black pepper

1. In a blender or in a large bowl, if using an immersion blender, combine the tomatoes, avocados, cucumber, bell pepper, yogurt, olive oil, cilantro, scallions, vinegar, and lime juice. Blend until smooth. If using a stand blender, you may need to blend in two or three batches.
2. Season with salt and pepper and blend to combine the flavors.
3. Chill in the refrigerator for 1 to 2 hours before serving. Serve cold.

Per Serving
calories: 392 | fat: 32g | protein: 6g
carbs: 20g | fiber: 9g | sodium: 335mg

Mushroom Barley Soup

Prep time: 5 minutes | Cook time: 25 minutes | Serves 6

2 tablespoons extra-virgin olive oil
1 cup chopped onion (about ½ medium onion)
1 cup chopped carrots (about 2 carrots)
5½ cups chopped mushrooms (about 12 ounces / 340 g)
6 cups low-sodium or no-salt-added
vegetable broth
1 cup uncooked pearled barley
¼ cup red wine
2 tablespoons tomato paste
4 sprigs fresh thyme or ½ teaspoon dried thyme
1 dried bay leaf
6 tablespoons grated Parmesan cheese

1. In a large stockpot over medium heat, heat the oil. Add the onion and carrots and cook for 5 minutes, stirring frequently. Turn up the heat to medium-high and add the mushrooms. Cook for 3 minutes, stirring frequently.
2. Add the broth, barley, wine, tomato paste, thyme, and bay leaf. Stir, cover the pot, and bring the soup to a boil. Once it's boiling, stir a few times, reduce the heat to medium-low, cover, and cook for another 12 to 15 minutes, until the barley is cooked through.
3. Remove the bay leaf and serve in soup bowls with 1 tablespoon of cheese sprinkled on top of each.

Per Serving
calories: 195 | fat: 4g | protein: 7g
carbs: 34g | fiber: 6g | sodium: 173mg

Red Lentil and Carrot Soup

Prep time: 10 minutes | Cook time: 20 minutes | Serves 6 to 8

1 cup red lentils, picked over and rinsed
½ cup long grain or basmati rice, rinsed
10 cups water
2 teaspoons salt
3 tablespoons extra-
virgin olive oil
1 large onion, finely chopped
2 cups carrots, finely diced
1 teaspoon turmeric
1 lemon, cut into wedges

1. In a large pot over medium heat, heat the lentils, rice, water, and salt. Bring to a simmer for 40 minutes, stirring occasionally.
2. In a small skillet over medium-low heat, cook the olive oil and onions for 5 minutes until the onions are golden brown.
3. Add the cooked onions, carrots, and turmeric to the soup and cook for 15 minutes, stirring occasionally.
4. Serve the soup with a big squeeze of lemon over the top and a lemon wedge on the side.

Per Serving
calories: 230 | fat: 7g | protein: 9g
carbs: 36g | fiber: 9g | sodium: 806mg

Chicken Provençal Soup

Prep time: 20 minutes | Cook time: 30 minutes | Serves 6 to 8

1 tablespoon extra-virgin olive oil
2 fennel bulbs, 2 tablespoons fronds minced, stalks discarded, bulbs halved, cored, and cut into ½-inch pieces
1 onion, chopped
1¾ teaspoons table salt
2 tablespoons tomato paste
4 garlic cloves, minced
1 tablespoon minced fresh thyme or 1 teaspoon dried
2 anchovy fillets, minced

7 cups water, divided
1 (14½-ounce / 411-g) can diced tomatoes, drained
2 carrots, peeled, halved lengthwise, and sliced ½ inch thick
2 (12-ounce / 340-g) bone-in split chicken breasts, trimmed
4 (5- to 7-ounce / 142- to 198-g) bone-in chicken thighs, trimmed
½ cup pitted brine-cured green olives, chopped
1 teaspoon grated orange zest

1. Using highest sauté function, heat oil in Instant Pot until shimmering. Add fennel pieces, onion, and salt and cook until vegetables are softened, about 5 minutes. Stir in tomato paste, garlic, thyme, and anchovies and cook until fragrant, about 30 seconds. Stir in 5 cups water, scraping up any browned bits, then stir in tomatoes and carrots. Nestle chicken breasts and thighs in pot.
2. Lock lid in place and close pressure release valve. Select high pressure cook function and cook for 20 minutes. Turn off Instant Pot and quick-release pressure. Carefully remove lid, allowing steam to escape away from you.
3. Transfer chicken to cutting board, let cool slightly, then shred into bite-size pieces using 2 forks; discard skin and bones.
4. Using wide, shallow spoon, skim excess fat from surface of soup. Stir chicken and any accumulated juices, olives, and remaining 2 cups water into soup and let sit until heated through, about 3 minutes. Stir in fennel fronds and orange zest, and season with salt and pepper to taste. Serve.

Per Serving

calories: 170 | fat: 5g | protein: 19g
carbs: 11g | fiber: 3g | sodium: 870mg

Paella Soup

Prep time: 5 minutes | Cook time: 25 minutes | Serves 6

1 cup frozen green peas
2 tablespoons extra-virgin olive oil
1 cup chopped onion (about ½ medium onion)
1½ cups coarsely chopped red bell pepper (about 1 large pepper)
1½ cups coarsely chopped green bell pepper (about 1 large pepper)
2 garlic cloves, chopped (about 1 teaspoon)
1 teaspoon ground turmeric

1 teaspoon dried thyme
2 teaspoons smoked paprika
2½ cups uncooked instant brown rice
2 cups low-sodium or no-salt-added chicken broth
2½ cups water
1 (28-ounce / 794-g) can low-sodium or no-salt-added crushed tomatoes
1 pound (454 g) fresh raw medium shrimp (or frozen raw shrimp completely thawed), shells and tails removed

1. Put the frozen peas on the counter to partially thaw as the soup is being prepared.
2. In a large stockpot over medium-high heat, heat the oil. Add the onion, red and green bell peppers, and garlic. Cook for 8 minutes, stirring occasionally. Add the turmeric, thyme, and smoked paprika, and cook for 2 minutes more, stirring often. Stir in the rice, broth, and water. Bring to a boil over high heat. Cover, reduce the heat to medium-low, and cook for 10 minutes.
3. Stir the peas, tomatoes, and shrimp into the soup. Cook for 4 to 6 minutes, until the shrimp is cooked, turning from gray to pink and white. The soup will be very thick, almost like stew, when ready to serve.

Per Serving

calories: 275 | fat: 5g | protein: 18g
carbs: 41g | fiber: 6g | sodium: 644mg

Thyme Carrot Soup with Parmesan
Prep time: 10 minutes | Cook time: 20 minutes | Serves 4

2 pounds (907 g) carrots, unpeeled, cut into ½-inch slices (about 6 cups)
2 tablespoons extra-virgin olive oil, divided
1 cup chopped onion (about ½ medium onion)
2 cups low-sodium or no-salt-added vegetable (or chicken) broth
2½ cups water
1 teaspoon dried thyme
¼ teaspoon crushed red pepper
¼ teaspoon kosher or sea salt
4 thin slices whole-grain bread
1/3 cup freshly grated Parmesan cheese (about 1 ounce / 28 g)

1. Place one oven rack about four inches below the broiler element. Place two large, rimmed baking sheets in the oven on any oven rack. Preheat the oven to 450°F (235°C).
2. In a large bowl, toss the carrots with 1 tablespoon of oil to coat. With oven mitts, carefully remove the baking sheets from the oven and evenly distribute the carrots on both sheets. Bake for 20 minutes, until the carrots are just fork tender, stirring once halfway through. The carrots will still be somewhat firm. Remove the carrots from the oven, and turn the oven to the high broil setting.
3. While the carrots are roasting, in a large stockpot over medium-high heat, heat 1 tablespoon of oil. Add the onion and cook for 5 minutes, stirring occasionally. Add the broth, water, thyme, crushed red pepper, and salt. Bring to a boil, cover, then remove the pan from the heat until the carrots have finished roasting.
4. Add the roasted carrots to the pot, and blend with an immersion blender (or use a regular blender—carefully pour in the hot soup in batches, then return the soup to the pot). Heat the soup for about 1 minute over medium-high heat, until warmed through.
5. Turn the oven to the high broil setting. Place the bread on the baking sheet. Sprinkle the cheese evenly across the slices of bread. Broil the bread 4 inches

below the heating element for 1 to 2 minutes, or until the cheese melts, watching carefully to prevent burning.
6. Cut the bread into bite-size croutons. Divide the soup evenly among four bowls, top each with the Parmesan croutons, and serve.

Per Serving
calories: 312 | fat: 6g | protein: 6g
carbs: 53g | fiber: 10g | sodium: 650mg

Pastina Chicken Soup
Prep time: 5 minutes | Cook time: 25 minutes | Serves 6

1 tablespoon extra-virgin olive oil
2 garlic cloves, minced (about 1 teaspoon)
3 cups packed chopped kale (center ribs removed)
1 cup minced carrots (about 2 carrots)
8 cups low-sodium or no-salt-added chicken (or vegetable) broth
¼ teaspoon kosher or sea salt
¼ teaspoon freshly ground black pepper
¾ cup (6 ounces / 170 g) uncooked acini de pepe or pastina pasta
2 cups shredded cooked chicken (about 12 ounces / 340 g)
3 tablespoons grated Parmesan cheese

1. In a large stockpot over medium heat, heat the oil. Add the garlic and cook for 30 seconds, stirring frequently. Add the kale and carrots and cook for 5 minutes, stirring occasionally.
2. Add the broth, salt, and pepper, and turn the heat to high. Bring the broth to a boil, and add the pasta. Lower the heat to medium and cook for 10 minutes, or until the pasta is cooked through, stirring every few minutes so the pasta doesn't stick to the bottom. Add the chicken, and cook for 2 more minutes to warm through.
3. Ladle the soup into six bowls, top each with ½ tablespoon of cheese, and serve.

Per Serving
calories: 275 | fat: 19g | protein: 16g
carbs: 11g | fiber: 2g | sodium: 298mg

Lentil and Chorizo Sausage Soup

Prep time: 15 minutes | Cook time: 18 minutes | Serves 6 to 8

1 tablespoon extra-virgin olive oil, plus extra for drizzling
8 ounces (227 g) Spanish-style chorizo sausage, quartered lengthwise and sliced thin
4 garlic cloves, minced
1½ teaspoons smoked paprika
5 cups water
1 pound (454 g) French green lentils, picked over and rinsed
4 cups chicken broth
1 tablespoon sherry vinegar, plus extra for seasoning
2 bay leaves
1 teaspoon table salt
1 large onion, peeled
2 carrots, peeled and halved crosswise
½ cup slivered almonds, toasted
½ cup minced fresh parsley

1. Using highest sauté function, heat oil in Instant Pot until shimmering. Add chorizo and cook until lightly browned, 3 to 5 minutes. Stir in garlic and paprika and cook until fragrant, about 30 seconds. Stir in water, scraping up any browned bits, then stir in lentils, broth, vinegar, bay leaves, and salt. Nestle onion and carrots into pot.
2. Lock lid in place and close pressure release valve. Select high pressure cook function and cook for 14 minutes. Turn off Instant Pot and quick-release pressure. Carefully remove lid, allowing steam to escape away from you.
3. Discard bay leaves. Using slotted spoon, transfer onion and carrots to food processor and process until smooth, about 1 minute, scraping down sides of bowl as needed. Stir vegetable mixture into lentils and season with salt, pepper, and extra vinegar to taste. Drizzle individual portions with extra oil, and sprinkle with almonds and parsley before serving.

Per Serving
calories: 360 | fat: 16g | protein: 21g
carbs: 29g | fiber: 7g | sodium: 950mg

Moroccan Lamb Lentil Soup

Prep time: 15 minutes | Cook time: 28 minutes | Serves 6 to 8

1 pound (454 g) lamb shoulder chops (blade or round bone), 1 to 1½ inches thick, trimmed and halved
¾ teaspoon table salt, divided
⅛ teaspoon pepper
1 tablespoon extra-virgin olive oil
1 onion, chopped fine
¼ cup harissa, plus extra for serving
1 tablespoon all-purpose flour
8 cups chicken broth
1 cup French green lentils, picked over and rinsed
1 (15-ounce / 425-g) can chickpeas, rinsed
2 tomatoes, cored and cut into ¼-inch pieces
½ cup chopped fresh cilantro

1. Pat lamb dry with paper towels and sprinkle with ¼ teaspoon salt and pepper. Using highest sauté function, heat oil in Instant Pot for 5 minutes (or until just smoking). Place lamb in pot and cook until well browned on first side, about 4 minutes; transfer to plate.
2. Add onion and remaining ½ teaspoon salt to fat left in pot and cook, using highest sauté function, until softened, about 5 minutes. Stir in harissa and flour and cook until fragrant, about 30 seconds. Slowly whisk in broth, scraping up any browned bits and smoothing out any lumps. Stir in lentils, then nestle lamb into multicooker and add any accumulated juices.
3. Lock lid in place and close pressure release valve. Select high pressure cook function and cook for 10 minutes. Turn off Instant Pot and quick-release pressure. Carefully remove lid, allowing steam to escape away from you.
4. Transfer lamb to cutting board, let cool slightly, then shred into bite-size pieces using 2 forks; discard excess fat and bones. Stir lamb and chickpeas into soup and let sit until heated through, about 3 minutes. Season with salt and pepper to taste. Top individual portions with tomatoes and sprinkle with cilantro. Serve, passing extra harissa separately.

Per Serving
calories: 300 | fat: 13g | protein: 22g
carbs: 24g | fiber: 6g | sodium: 940mg

Pasta Bean Soup
Prep time: 5 minutes | Cook time: 25 minutes | Serves 6

2 tablespoons extra-virgin olive oil
½ cup chopped onion (about ¼ onion)
3 garlic cloves, minced (about 1½ teaspoons)
1 tablespoon minced fresh rosemary or 1 teaspoon dried rosemary
¼ teaspoon crushed red pepper
4 cups low-sodium or no-salt-added vegetable broth
2 (15½-ounce / 439-g) cans cannellini, great

northern, or light kidney beans, undrained
1 (28-ounce / 794-g) can low-sodium or no-salt-added crushed tomatoes
2 tablespoons tomato paste
8 ounces (227 g) uncooked short pasta, such as ditalini, tubetti, or elbows
6 tablespoons grated Parmesan cheese (about 1½ ounces / 43 g)

1. In a large stockpot over medium heat, heat the oil. Add the onion and cook for 4 minutes, stirring frequently. Add the garlic, rosemary, and crushed red pepper. Cook for 1 minute, stirring frequently. Add the broth, canned beans with their liquid, tomatoes, and tomato paste. Simmer for 5 minutes.
2. To thicken the soup, carefully transfer 2 cups to a blender. Purée, then stir it back into the pot.
3. Bring the soup to a boil over high heat. Mix in the pasta, and lower the heat to a simmer. Cook the pasta for the amount of time recommended on the box, stirring every few minutes to prevent the pasta from sticking to the pot. Taste the pasta to make sure it is cooked through (it could take a few more minutes than the recommended cooking time, since it's cooking with other ingredients).
4. Ladle the soup into bowls, top each with 1 tablespoon of grated cheese, and serve.

Per Serving
calories: 583 | fat: 6g | protein: 32g | carbs: 103g | fiber: 29g | sodium: 234mg

White Bean and Carrot Soup
Prep time: 10 minutes | Cook time: 20 minutes | Serves 6

3 tablespoons extra-virgin olive oil
1 large onion, finely chopped
3 large garlic cloves, minced
2 cups carrots, diced
2 cups celery, diced

2 (15-ounce / 425-g) cans white beans, rinsed and drained
8 cups vegetable broth
1 teaspoon salt
½ teaspoon freshly ground black pepper

1. In a large pot over medium heat, cook the olive oil, onion, and garlic for 2 to 3 minutes.
2. Add the carrots and celery, and cook for another 3 to 5 minutes, stirring occasionally.
3. Add the beans, broth, salt, and pepper. Stir and let simmer for 15 to 17 minutes, stirring occasionally. Serve warm.

Per Serving
calories: 244 | fat: 7g | protein: 9g | carbs: 36g | fiber: 10g | sodium: 1160mg

Almond and Cauliflower Gazpacho

Prep time: 10 minutes | Cook time: 16 minutes | Serves 4 to 6

1 cup raw almonds
½ teaspoon salt
½ cup extra-virgin olive oil, plus 1 tablespoon, divided
1 small white onion, minced
1 small head cauliflower, stalk removed and

broken into florets (about 3 cups)
2 garlic cloves, finely minced
2 cups chicken or vegetable stock or broth, plus more if needed
1 tablespoon red wine vinegar
¼ teaspoon freshly ground black pepper

1. Bring a small pot of water to a boil. Add the almonds to the water and boil for 1 minute, being careful to not boil longer or the almonds will become soggy. Drain in a colander and run under cold water. Pat dry and, using your fingers, squeeze the meat of each almond out of its skin. Discard the skins.
2. In a food processor or blender, blend together the almonds and salt. With the processor running, drizzle in ½ cup extra-virgin olive oil, scraping down the sides as needed. Set the almond paste aside.
3. In a large stockpot, heat the remaining 1 tablespoon olive oil over medium-high heat. Add the onion and sauté until golden, 3 to 4 minutes. Add the cauliflower florets and sauté for another 3 to 4 minutes. Add the garlic and sauté for 1 minute more.
4. Add 2 cups stock and bring to a boil. Cover, reduce the heat to medium-low, and simmer the vegetables until tender, 8 to 10 minutes. Remove from the heat and allow to cool slightly.
5. Add the vinegar and pepper. Using an immersion blender, blend until smooth. Alternatively, you can blend in a stand blender, but you may need to divide the mixture into two or three batches. With the blender running, add the almond paste and blend until smooth, adding extra stock if the soup is too thick.
6. Serve warm, or chill in refrigerator at least 4 to 6 hours to serve a cold gazpacho.

Per Serving
calories: 505 | fat: 45g | protein: 10g | carbs: 10g | fiber: 5g | sodium: 484mg

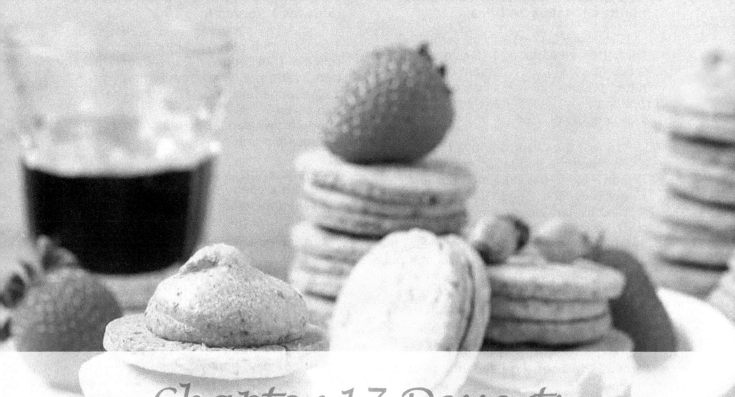
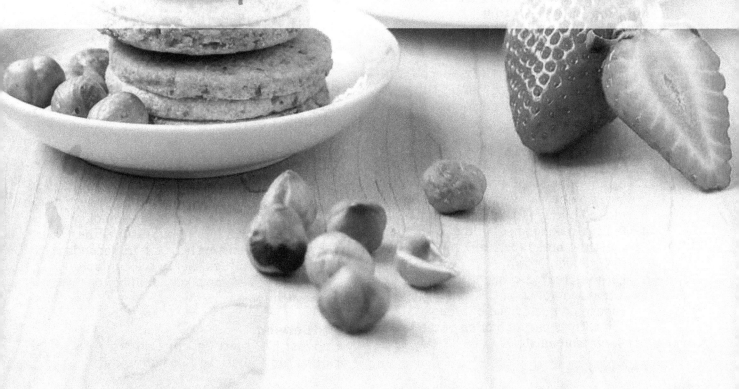

Chapter 17 Desserts

Vanilla Cake Bites

Prep time: 10 minutes | Cook time: 45 minutes | Makes 24 bites

1 (12-ounce / 340-g) box butter cake mix
½ cup (1 stick) butter, melted (optional)
3 large eggs, divided
1 cup sugar
1 (8-ounce / 227-g) cream cheese
1 teaspoon vanilla extract

1. Preheat the oven to 350ºF (180ºC).
2. To make the first layer, in a medium bowl, blend the cake mix, butter (if desired), and 1 egg. Then, pour the mixture into the prepared pan.
3. In a separate bowl, to make layer 2, mix together sugar, cream cheese, the remaining 2 eggs, and vanilla and pour this gently over the first layer. Bake for 45 to 50 minutes and allow to cool.
4. Cut the cake into 24 small squares.

Per Serving

calories: 160 | fat: 8g | protein: 2g
carbs: 20g | fiber: 0g | sodium: 156mg

Fig Crostini with Mascarpone

Prep time: 10 minutes | Cook time: 10 minutes | Serves 6 to 8

1 long French baguette
4 tablespoons (½ stick) salted butter, melted (optional)
1 (8-ounce / 227-
g) tub mascarpone cheese
1 (12-ounce / 340-g) jar fig jam or preserves

1. Preheat the oven to 350ºF (180ºC).
2. Slice the bread into ¼-inch-thick slices.
3. Arrange the sliced bread on a baking sheet and brush each slice with the melted butter (if desired).
4. Put the baking sheet in the oven and toast the bread for 5 to 7 minutes, just until golden brown.
5. Let the bread cool slightly. Spread about a teaspoon or so of the mascarpone cheese on each piece of bread.
6. Top with a teaspoon or so of the jam. Serve immediately.

Per Serving

calories: 445 | fat: 24g | protein: 3g
carbs: 48g | fiber: 5g | sodium: 314mg

Apple Pie Pockets

Prep time: 5 minutes | Cook time: 15 minutes | Serves 6

1 organic puff pastry, rolled out, at room temperature
1 Gala apple, peeled and sliced
¼ cup brown sugar
⅛ teaspoon ground
cinnamon
⅛ teaspoon ground cardamom
Nonstick cooking spray
Honey, for topping

1. Preheat the oven to 350ºF (180ºC).
2. Cut the pastry dough into 4 even discs. Peel and slice the apple. In a small bowl, toss the slices with brown sugar, cinnamon, and cardamom.
3. Spray a muffin tin very well with nonstick cooking spray. Be sure to spray only the muffin holders you plan to use.
4. Once sprayed, line the bottom of the muffin tin with the dough and place 1 or 2 broken apple slices on top. Fold the remaining dough over the apple and drizzle with honey.
5. Bake for 15 minutes or until brown and bubbly.

Per Serving

calories: 250 | fat: 15g | protein: 3g
carbs: 30g | fiber: 1g | sodium: 98mg

Berry and Honey Compote

Prep time: 5 minutes | Cook time: 2 to 5 minutes | Serves 2 to 3

½ cup honey
¼ cup fresh berries
2 tablespoons grated orange zest

1. In a small saucepan, heat the honey, berries, and orange zest over medium-low heat for 2 to 5 minutes, until the sauce thickens, or heat for 15 seconds in the microwave. Serve the compote drizzled over pancakes, muffins, or French toast.

Per Serving

calories: 272 | fat: 0g | protein: 1g
carbs: 74g | fiber: 1g | sodium: 4mg

Sesame Seed Cookies

Prep time: 10 minutes | Cook time: 15 minutes | Makes 14 to 16 cookies

1 cup sesame seeds, hulled	stick) salted butter, softened (optional)
1 cup sugar	2 large eggs
8 tablespoons (1	1¼ cups flour

1. Preheat the oven to 350ºF (180ºC). Toast the sesame seeds on a baking sheet for 3 minutes. Set aside and let cool.
2. Using a mixer, cream together the sugar and butter (if desired).
3. Add the eggs one at a time until well-blended.
4. Add the flour and toasted sesame seeds and mix until well-blended.
5. Drop spoonfuls of cookie dough onto a baking sheet and form them into round balls, about 1-inch in diameter, similar to a walnut.
6. Put in the oven and bake for 5 to 7 minutes or until golden brown.
7. Let the cookies cool and enjoy.

Per Serving
calories: 218 | fat: 12g | protein: 4g
carbs: 25g | fiber: 2g | sodium: 58mg

Buttery Almond Cookies

Prep time: 5 minutes | Cook time: 10 minutes | Serves 4 to 6

½ cup sugar	1½ cups all-purpose flour
8 tablespoons (1 stick) room temperature salted butter (optional)	1 cup ground almonds or almond flour
1 large egg	

1. Preheat the oven to 375ºF (190ºC).
2. Using a mixer, cream together the sugar and butter (if desired).
3. Add the egg and mix until combined.
4. Alternately add the flour and ground almonds, ½ cup at a time, while the mixer is on slow.
5. Once everything is combined, line a baking sheet with parchment paper. Drop a tablespoon of dough on the baking sheet, keeping the cookies at least 2 inches apart.

6. Put the baking sheet in the oven and bake just until the cookies start to turn brown around the edges, about 5 to 7 minutes.

Per Serving
calories: 604 | fat: 36g | protein: 11g
carbs: 63g | fiber: 4g | sodium: 181mg

Strawberry Shortbread Cookies

Prep time: 20 minutes | Cook time: 10 minutes | Makes 3 dozen cookies

2 cups cornstarch	⅔ cup sugar
1½ cups all-purpose flour	4 large egg yolks
2 teaspoons baking powder	2 tablespoons brandy
1 teaspoon baking soda	1 teaspoon vanilla extract
1 cup (2 sticks) cold butter, cut into 1-inch cubes (optional)	½ teaspoon salt
	2 cups strawberry preserves
	Confectioners' sugar, for sprinkling

1. In a bowl, combine the cornstarch, flour, baking powder, and baking soda and mix together. Using your hands or 2 forks, mix the butter (if desired) and sugar just until combined, with small pieces of butter remaining.
2. Add the egg yolks, brandy, vanilla, and salt, stirring slowly until all ingredients are blended together. If you have a stand mixer, you can mix these ingredients together with the paddle attachment and then finish mixing by hand, but it is not required.
3. Wrap the dough in plastic wrap and place in a resealable plastic bag for at least 1 hour.
4. Preheat the oven to 350ºF (180ºC).
5. Roll the dough to ¼-inch thickness and cut, placing 12 cookies on a sheet. Bake the sheets one at a time on the top rack of the oven for 12 to 14 minutes.
6. Let the cookies cool completely and top with about 1 tablespoon of strawberry preserves.
7. Sprinkle with confectioners' sugar.

Per Serving
calories: 157 | fat: 6g | protein: 1g
carbs: 26g | fiber: 0g | sodium: 132mg

Creamy Rice Pudding
Prep time: 5 minutes | Cook time: 45 minutes | Serves 6

1¼ cups long-grain rice	1 tablespoon rose water or orange blossom water
5 cups unsweetened almond milk	1 teaspoon cinnamon
1 cup sugar	

1. Rinse the rice under cold water for 30 seconds.
2. Put the rice, milk, and sugar in a large pot. Bring to a gentle boil while continually stirring.
3. Turn the heat down to low and let simmer for 40 to 45 minutes, stirring every 3 to 4 minutes so that the rice does not stick to the bottom of the pot.
4. Add the rose water at the end and simmer for 5 minutes.
5. Divide the pudding into 6 bowls. Sprinkle the top with cinnamon. Cool for at least 1 hour before serving. Store in the fridge.

Per Serving
calories: 323 | fat: 7g | protein: 9g
carbs: 56g | fiber: 1g | sodium: 102mg

Cream Cheese and Ricotta Cheesecake
Prep time: 5 minutes | Cook time: 1 hour | Serves 8 to 10

2 (8-ounce / 227-g) packages full-fat cream cheese	sugar
	1 tablespoon lemon zest
1 (16-ounce / 454-g) container full-fat ricotta cheese	5 large eggs
	Nonstick cooking spray
1½ cups granulated	

1. Preheat the oven to 350ºF (180ºC).
2. Using a mixer, blend together the cream cheese and ricotta cheese.
3. Blend in the sugar and lemon zest.
4. Blend in the eggs; drop in 1 egg at a time, blend for 10 seconds, and repeat.
5. Line a 9-inch springform pan with parchment paper and nonstick spray. Wrap the bottom of the pan with foil. Pour the cheesecake batter into the pan.

6. To make a water bath, get a baking or roasting pan larger than the cheesecake pan. Fill the roasting pan about ⅓ of the way up with warm water. Put the cheesecake pan into the water bath. Put the whole thing in the oven and let the cheesecake bake for 1 hour.
7. After baking is complete, remove the cheesecake pan from the water bath and remove the foil. Let the cheesecake cool for 1 hour on the countertop. Then put it in the fridge to cool for at least 3 hours before serving.

Per Serving
calories: 489 | fat: 31g | protein: 15g
carbs: 42g | fiber: 0g | sodium: 264mg

Grilled Fruit Skewers
Prep time: 15 minutes | Cook time: 10 minutes | Serves 2

⅔ cup prepared labneh, or, if making your own, ⅔ cup full-fat plain Greek yogurt	Pinch salt
	3 cups fresh fruit cut into 2-inch chunks (pineapple, cantaloupe, nectarines, strawberries, plums, or mango)
2 tablespoons honey	
1 teaspoon vanilla extract	

1. If making your own labneh, place a colander over a bowl and line it with cheesecloth. Place the Greek yogurt in the cheesecloth and wrap it up. Put the bowl in the refrigerator and let sit for at least 12 to 24 hours, until it's thick like soft cheese.
2. Mix honey, vanilla, and salt into labneh. Stir well to combine and set it aside.
3. Heat the grill to medium (about 300ºF / 150ºC) and oil the grill grate. Alternatively, you can cook these on the stovetop in a heavy grill pan (cast iron works well).
4. Thread the fruit onto skewers and grill for 4 minutes on each side, or until fruit is softened and has grill marks on each side.
5. Serve the fruit with labneh to dip.

Per Serving
calories: 292 | fat: 6g | protein: 5g
carbs: 60g | fiber: 4g | sodium: 131mg

Cranberry Orange Loaf

Prep time: 20 minutes | Cook time: 45 minutes | Makes 1 loaf

Dough:

3 cups all-purpose flour
1 (¼-ounce / 7-g) package quick-rise yeast
½ teaspoon salt
⅛ teaspoon ground cinnamon
⅛ teaspoon ground cardamom
½ cup water
½ cup almond milk
⅓ cup butter, cubed (optional)

Cranberry Filling:

1 (12-ounce / 340-g) can cranberry sauce
½ cup chopped walnuts
2 tablespoons grated orange zest
2 tablespoons orange juice

1. In a large bowl, combine the flour, yeast, salt, cinnamon, and cardamom.
2. In a small pot, heat the water, almond milk, and butter (if desired) over medium-high heat. Once it boils, reduce the heat to medium-low. Simmer for 10 to 15 minutes, until the liquid thickens.
3. Pour the liquid ingredients into the dry ingredients and, using a wooden spoon or spatula, mix the dough until it forms a ball in the bowl.
4. Put the dough in a greased bowl, cover tightly with a kitchen towel, and set aside for 1 hour.
5. To make the cranberry filling: In a medium bowl, mix the cranberry sauce with walnuts, orange zest, and orange juice in a large bowl.
6. Assemble the Bread
7. Roll out the dough to about a 1-inch-thick and 10-by-7-inch-wide rectangle.
8. Spread the cranberry filling evenly on the surface of the rolled-out dough, leaving a 1-inch border around the edges. Starting with the long side, tuck the dough under with your fingertips and roll up the dough tightly. Place the rolled-up dough in an "S" shape in a bread pan.
9. Allow the bread to rise again, about 30 to 40 minutes.
10. Preheat the oven to 350ºF (180ºC).
11. Bake in a preheated oven, 45 minutes.

Per Serving

calories: 483 | fat: 15g | protein: 8g
carbs: 79g | fiber: 4g | sodium: 232mg

Honey Walnut Baklava

Prep time: 30 minutes | Cook time: 1 hour | Serves 6 to 8

2 cups very finely chopped walnuts or pecans
1 teaspoon cinnamon
1 cup (2 sticks) unsalted butter, melted (optional)
1 (16-ounce / 454-g) package phyllo dough, thawed
1 (12-ounce / 340-g) jar honey

1. Preheat the oven to 350ºF (180ºC).
2. In a bowl, combine the chopped nuts and cinnamon.
3. Using a brush, butter the sides and bottom of a 9-by-13-inch inch baking dish.
4. Remove the phyllo dough from the package and cut it to the size of the baking dish using a sharp knife.
5. Place one sheet of phyllo dough on the bottom of the dish, brush with butter, and repeat until you have 8 layers.
6. Sprinkle ⅓ cup of the nut mixture over the phyllo layers. Top with a sheet of phyllo dough, butter that sheet, and repeat until you have 4 sheets of buttered phyllo dough.
7. Sprinkle ⅓ cup of the nut mixture for another layer of nuts. Repeat the layering of nuts and 4 sheets of buttered phyllo until all the nut mixture is gone. The last layer should be 8 buttered sheets of phyllo.
8. Before you bake, cut the baklava into desired shapes; traditionally this is diamonds, triangles, or squares.
9. Bake the baklava for 1 hour or until the top layer is golden brown.
10. While the baklava is baking, heat the honey in a pan just until it is warm and easy to pour.
11. Once the baklava is done baking, immediately pour the honey evenly over the baklava and let it absorb it, about 20 minutes. Serve warm or at room temperature.

Per Serving

calories: 754 | fat: 46g | protein: 8g
carbs: 77g | fiber: 3g | sodium: 33mg

Pound Cake with Citrus Glaze

Prep time: 10 minutes | Cook time: 45 minutes | Serves 8

Cake:

Nonstick cooking spray
1 cup sugar
$1/_3$ cup extra-virgin olive oil
1 cup unsweetened almond milk

1 lemon, zested and juiced
2 cups all-purpose flour
1 teaspoon baking soda
1 teaspoon salt

Glaze:

1 cup powdered sugar
1 to 2 tablespoons freshly squeezed

lemon juice
½ teaspoon vanilla extract

Make the Cake

1. Preheat the oven to 350ºF (180ºC). Line a 9-inch loaf pan with parchment paper and coat the paper with nonstick cooking spray.
2. In a large bowl, whisk together the sugar and olive oil until creamy. Whisk in the milk and lemon juice and zest. Let it stand for 5 to 7 minutes.
3. In a medium bowl, combine the flour, baking soda, and salt. Fold the dry ingredients into the milk mixture and stir just until incorporated.
4. Pour the batter into the prepared pan and smooth the top. Bake until a toothpick or skewer inserted into the middle comes out clean with a few crumbs attached, about 45 minutes.
5. Remove the cake from the oven and cool for at least 10 minutes in the pan. Transfer to a cooling rack placed over a baking sheet and cool completely.

Make the Glaze

1. In a small bowl, whisk together the powdered sugar, lemon juice, and vanilla until smooth. Pour the glaze over the cooled cake, allowing the excess to drip off the cake onto the baking sheet beneath.

Per Serving

calories: 347 | fat: 9g | protein: 4g
carbs: 64g | fiber: 1g | sodium: 481mg

Pomegranate and Quinoa Dark Chocolate Bark

Prep time: 5 minutes | Cook time: 13 minutes | Serves 6

Nonstick cooking spray
½ cup uncooked tricolor or regular quinoa
½ teaspoon kosher or sea salt

8 ounces (227 g) dark chocolate or 1 cup dark chocolate chips
½ cup fresh pomegranate seeds

1. In a medium saucepan coated with nonstick cooking spray over medium heat, toast the uncooked quinoa for 2 to 3 minutes, stirring frequently. Do not let the quinoa burn. Remove the pan from the stove, and mix in the salt. Set aside 2 tablespoons of the toasted quinoa to use for the topping.
2. Break the chocolate into large pieces, and put it in a gallon-size zip-top plastic bag. Using a metal ladle or a meat pounder, pound the chocolate until broken into smaller pieces. (If using chocolate chips, you can skip this step.) Dump the chocolate out of the bag into a medium, microwave-safe bowl and heat for 1 minute on high in the microwave. Stir until the chocolate is completely melted. Mix the toasted quinoa (except the topping you set aside) into the melted chocolate.
3. Line a large, rimmed baking sheet with parchment paper. Pour the chocolate mixture onto the sheet and spread it evenly until the entire pan is covered. Sprinkle the remaining 2 tablespoons of quinoa and the pomegranate seeds on top. Using a spatula or the back of a spoon, press the quinoa and the pomegranate seeds into the chocolate.
4. Freeze the mixture for 10 to 15 minutes, or until set. Remove the bark from the freezer, and break it into about 2-inch jagged pieces. Store in a sealed container or zip-top plastic bag in the refrigerator until ready to serve.

Per Serving

calories: 268 | fat: 11g | protein: 4g
carbs: 37g | fiber: 2g | sodium: 360mg

Orange Mug Cake

Prep time: 10 minutes | Cook time: 2 minutes | Serves 2

6 tablespoons flour
2 tablespoons sugar
½ teaspoon baking powder
Pinch salt
1 teaspoon orange zest
1 egg
2 tablespoons olive oil

2 tablespoons freshly squeezed orange juice
2 tablespoons unsweetened almond milk
½ teaspoon orange extract
½ teaspoon vanilla extract

1. In a small bowl, combine the flour, sugar, baking powder, salt, and orange zest.
2. In a separate bowl, whisk together the egg, olive oil, orange juice, milk, orange extract, and vanilla extract.
3. Pour the dry ingredients into the wet ingredients and stir to combine. The batter will be thick.
4. Divide the mixture into two small mugs that hold at least 6 ounces / 170 g each, or 1 (12-ounce / 340-g) mug.
5. Microwave each mug separately. The small ones should take about 60 seconds, and one large mug should take about 90 seconds, but microwaves can vary. The cake will be done when it pulls away from the sides of the mug.

Per Serving
calories: 302 | fat: 17g | protein: 6g
carbs: 33g | fiber: 1g | sodium: 117mg

Baked Pears with Mascarpone Cheese

Prep time: 10 minutes | Cook time: 20 minutes | Serves 2

2 ripe pears, peeled
1 tablespoon plus 2 teaspoons honey, divided
1 teaspoon vanilla, divided
¼ teaspoon ginger

¼ teaspoon ground coriander
¼ cup minced walnuts
¼ cup mascarpone cheese
Pinch salt

1. Preheat the oven to 350ºF (180ºC) and set the rack to the middle position. Grease a small baking dish.
2. Cut the pears in half lengthwise. Using a spoon, scoop out the core from each piece. Place the pears with the cut side up in the baking dish.
3. Combine 1 tablespoon of honey, ½ teaspoon of vanilla, ginger, and coriander in a small bowl. Pour this mixture evenly over the pear halves.
4. Sprinkle walnuts over the pear halves.
5. Bake for 20 minutes, or until the pears are golden and you're able to pierce them easily with a knife.
6. While the pears are baking, mix the mascarpone cheese with the remaining 2 teaspoons honey, ½ teaspoon of vanilla, and a pinch of salt. Stir well to combine.
7. Divide the mascarpone among the warm pear halves and serve.

Per Serving
calories: 307 | fat: 16g | protein: 4g
carbs: 43g | fiber: 6g | sodium: 89mg

Chocolate Chia Seeds Pudding

Prep time: 5 minutes | Cook time: 5 minutes | Serves 4

2 cups heavy cream
¼ cup unsweetened cocoa powder
1 teaspoon almond extract or vanilla

extract
½ or 1 teaspoon ground cinnamon
¼ teaspoon salt
½ cup chia seeds

1. In a saucepan, heat the heavy cream over medium-low heat to just below a simmer. Remove from the heat and allow to cool slightly.
2. In a blender or large bowl, if using an immersion blender, combine the warmed heavy cream, cocoa powder, almond extract, cinnamon, and salt and blend until the cocoa is well incorporated.
3. Stir in the chia seeds and let sit for 15 minutes.
4. Divide the mixture evenly between ramekins or small glass bowls and refrigerate at least 6 hours, or until set. Serve chilled.

Per Serving
calories: 561 | fat: 52g | protein: 8g
carbs: 19g | fiber: 12g | sodium: 187mg

Quick Marzipan Fat Bomb
Prep time: 5 minutes | Cook time: 0 minutes | Serves 8

1½ cup finely ground almond flour
½ to 1 cup powdered sugar-free sweetener of choice

2 teaspoons almond extract
½ cup light fruity extra-virgin olive oil or avocado oil

1. Add the almond flour and sweetener to a food processor and run until the mixture is very finely ground.
2. Add the almond extract and pulse until combined. With the processor running, stream in olive oil until the mixture starts to form a large ball. Turn off the food processor.
3. Using your hands, form the marzipan into eight (1-inch) diameter balls, pressing to hold the mixture together. Store in an airtight container in the refrigerator for up to 2 weeks.

Per Serving (1 fat bomb)
calories: 157 | fat: 16g | protein: 2g
carbs: 0g | fiber: 0g | sodium: 0mg

Pomegranate Blueberry Granita
Prep time: 5 minutes | Cook time: 10 minutes | Serves 2

1 cup frozen wild blueberries
1 cup pomegranate or pomegranate

blueberry juice
¼ cup sugar
¼ cup water

1. Combine the frozen blueberries and pomegranate juice in a saucepan and bring to a boil. Reduce the heat and simmer for 5 minutes, or until the blueberries start to break down.
2. While the juice and berries are cooking, combine the sugar and water in a small microwave-safe bowl. Microwave for 60 seconds, or until it comes to a rolling boil. Stir to make sure all of the sugar is dissolved and set the syrup aside.
3. Combine the blueberry mixture and the sugar syrup in a blender and blend for 1 minute, or until the fruit is completely puréed.

4. Pour the mixture into an 8-by-8-inch baking pan or a similar-sized bowl. The liquid should come about ½ inch up the sides. Let the mixture cool for 30 minutes, and then put it into the freezer.
5. Every 30 minutes for the next 2 hours, scrape the granita with a fork to keep it from freezing solid.
6. Serve it after 2 hours, or store it in a covered container in the freezer.

Per Serving
calories: 214 | fat: 0g | protein: 1g
carbs: 54g | fiber: 2g | sodium: 15mg

Summer Strawberry Panna Cotta
Prep time: 10 minutes | Cook time: 5 minutes | Serves 4

2 tablespoons warm water
2 teaspoons gelatin powder
2 cups heavy cream
1 cup sliced strawberries, plus more for garnish

1 to 2 tablespoons sugar-free sweetener of choice (optional)
1½ teaspoons pure vanilla extract
4 to 6 fresh mint leaves, for garnish (optional)

1. Pour the warm water into a small bowl. Sprinkle the gelatin over the water and stir well to dissolve. Allow the mixture to sit for 10 minutes.
2. In a blender or a large bowl, if using an immersion blender, combine the cream, strawberries, sweetener (if using), and vanilla. Blend until the mixture is smooth and the strawberries are well puréed.
3. Transfer the mixture to a saucepan and heat over medium-low heat until just below a simmer. Remove from the heat and cool for 5 minutes.
4. Whisking constantly, add in the gelatin mixture until smooth. Divide the custard between ramekins or small glass bowls, cover and refrigerate until set, 4 to 6 hours.
5. Serve chilled, garnishing with additional sliced strawberries or mint leaves (if using).

Per Serving
calories: 431 | fat: 43g | protein: 4g
carbs: 7g | fiber: 1g | sodium: 49mg

Orange Almond Cupcakes

Prep time: 10 minutes | Cook time: 15 minutes | Makes 6 cupcakes

1 large egg
2 tablespoons powdered sugar-free sweetener (such as stevia or monk fruit extract)
½ cup extra-virgin olive oil
1 teaspoon almond extract
Zest of 1 orange
1 cup almond flour
¾ teaspoon baking powder
⅛ teaspoon salt
1 tablespoon freshly squeezed orange juice

1. Preheat the oven to 350ºF (180ºC). Place muffin liners into 6 cups of a muffin tin.
2. In a large bowl, whisk together the egg and powdered sweetener. Add the olive oil, almond extract, and orange zest and whisk to combine well.
3. In a small bowl, whisk together the almond flour, baking powder, and salt. Add to wet ingredients along with the orange juice and stir until just combined.
4. Divide the batter evenly into 6 muffin cups and bake until a toothpick inserted in the center of the cupcake comes out clean, 15 to 18 minutes.
5. Remove from the oven and cool for 5 minutes in the tin before transferring to a wire rack to cool completely.

Per Serving
calories: 211 | fat: 21g | protein: 3g
carbs: 2g | fiber: 0g | sodium: 105mg

Ricotta Pumpkin Cheesecake

Prep time: 10 minutes | Cook time: 40 minutes | Serves 10 to 12

1 cup almond flour
½ cup butter, melted (optional)
1 (14½-ounce / 411-g) can pumpkin purée
8 ounces (227 g) cream cheese, at room temperature
½ cup whole-milk
Ricotta cheese
½ to ¾ cup sugar-free sweetener
4 large eggs
2 teaspoons vanilla extract
2 teaspoons pumpkin pie spice
Whipped cream, for garnish (optional)

1. Preheat the oven to 350ºF (180ºC). Line the bottom of a 9-inch springform pan with parchment paper.
2. In a small bowl, combine the almond flour and melted butter (if desired) with a fork until well combined. Using your fingers, press the mixture into the bottom of the prepared pan.
3. In a large bowl, beat together the pumpkin purée, cream cheese, ricotta, and sweetener using an electric mixer on medium.
4. Add the eggs, one at a time, beating after each addition. Stir in the vanilla and pumpkin pie spice until just combined.
5. Pour the mixture over the crust and bake until set, 40 to 45 minutes.
6. Allow to cool to room temperature. Refrigerate for at least 6 hours before serving.
7. Serve chilled, garnishing with whipped cream, if desired.

Per Serving
calories: 242 | fat: 22g | protein: 7g
carbs: 5g | fiber: 1g | sodium: 178mg

Mixed-Berries, Pecans and Oat Crumbles

Prep time: 5 minutes | Cook time: 30 minutes | Serves 2

1½ cups frozen mixed berries, thawed
1 tablespoon butter,
softened (optional)
1 tablespoon sugar
¼ cup pecans
¼ cup oats

1. Preheat the oven to 350ºF (180ºC) and set the rack to the middle position.
2. Divide the berries between 2 (8-ounce) ramekins
3. In a food processor, combine the butter (if desired), sugar, pecans, and oats, and pulse a few times, until the mixture resembles damp sand.
4. Divide the crumble topping over the berries.
5. Place the ramekins on a sheet pan and bake for 30 minutes, or until the top is golden and the berries are bubbling.

Per Serving
calories: 267 | fat: 16g | protein: 4g
carbs: 27g | fiber: 6g | sodium: 43mg

Blueberry, Pecan, and Oat Crisp

Prep time: 10 minutes | Cook time: 20 minutes | Serves 4

2 tablespoons coconut oil, melted, plus more for greasing
4 cups fresh blueberries
Juice of ½ lemon
2 teaspoons lemon zest

¼ cup maple syrup
1 cup gluten-free rolled oats
½ cup chopped pecans
½ teaspoon ground cinnamon
Sea salt, to taste

1. Preheat the oven to 350°F (180°C). Grease a baking sheet with coconut oil.
2. Combine the blueberries, lemon juice and zest, and maple syrup in a bowl. Stir to mix well, then spread the mixture on the baking sheet.
3. Combine the remaining ingredients in a small bowl. Stir to mix well. Pour the mixture over the blueberries mixture.
4. Bake in the preheated oven for 20 minutes or until the oats are golden brown.
5. Serve immediately with spoons.

Per Serving

calories: 496 | fat: 33g | protein: 5g
carbs: 51g | fiber: 7g | sodium: 41mg

Olive Oil Almond Cake

Prep time: 10 minutes | Cook time: 12 minutes | Serves 4

Olive oil cooking spray
1½ cups whole wheat flour, plus more for dusting
3 eggs
⅓ cup honey
½ cup olive oil
½ cup unsweetened

almond milk
½ teaspoon vanilla extract
½ teaspoon almond extract
1 teaspoon baking powder
½ teaspoon salt

1. Preheat the air fryer to 380°F (193°C). Lightly coat the interior of an 8-by-8-inch baking dish with olive oil cooking spray and a dusting of whole wheat flour. Knock out any excess flour.
2. In a large bowl, beat the eggs and honey until smooth.

3. Slowly mix in the olive oil, then the almond milk, and finally the vanilla and almond extracts until combined.
4. In a separate bowl, whisk together the flour, baking powder, and salt.
5. Slowly incorporate the dry ingredients into the wet ingredients with a rubber spatula until combined, making sure to scrape down the sides of the bowl as you mix.
6. Pour the batter into the prepared pan and place it in the air fryer. Bake for 12 to 15 minutes, or until a toothpick inserted in the center comes out clean.

Per Serving

calories: 546 | fat: 31g | protein: 12g
carbs: 58g | fiber: 3g | sodium: 361mg

Avocados Chocolate Pudding

Prep time: 10 minutes | Cook time: 0 minutes | Serves 4

2 ripe avocados, halved and pitted
¼ cup unsweetened cocoa powder
¼ cup heavy whipping cream, plus more if needed
2 teaspoons vanilla extract

1 to 2 teaspoons liquid stevia or monk fruit extract (optional)
½ teaspoon ground cinnamon (optional)
¼ teaspoon salt
Whipped cream, for serving (optional)

1. Using a spoon, scoop out the ripe avocado into a blender or large bowl, if using an immersion blender. Mash well with a fork.
2. Add the cocoa powder, heavy whipping cream, vanilla, sweetener (if using), cinnamon (if using), and salt. Blend well until smooth and creamy, adding additional cream, 1 tablespoon at a time, if the mixture is too thick.
3. Cover and refrigerate for at least 1 hour before serving. Serve chilled with additional whipped cream, if desired.

Per Serving

calories: 230 | fat: 21g | protein: 3g
carbs: 10g | fiber: 5g | sodium: 163mg

Lemon Fool with Honey Drizzled

Prep time: 10 minutes | Cook time: 2 minutes | Serves 4

1 cup 2% plain Greek yogurt
1 medium lemon
¼ cup cold water
1½ teaspoons cornstarch
3½ tablespoons honey, divided
⅔ cup heavy (whipping) cream
Fresh fruit and mint leaves, for serving (optional)

1. Place a large glass bowl and the metal beaters from your electric mixer in the refrigerator to chill. Add the yogurt to a medium glass bowl, and place that bowl in the refrigerator to chill as well.
2. Using a Microplane or citrus zester, zest the lemon into a medium, microwave-safe bowl. Halve the lemon, and squeeze 1 tablespoon of lemon juice into the bowl. Add the water and cornstarch, and stir well. Whisk in 3 tablespoons of honey. Microwave the lemon mixture on high for 1 minute; stir and microwave for an additional 10 to 30 seconds, until the mixture is thick and bubbling.
3. Remove the bowl of yogurt from the refrigerator, and whisk in the warm lemon mixture. Place the yogurt back in the refrigerator.
4. Remove the large chilled bowl and the beaters from the refrigerator. Assemble your electric mixer with the chilled beaters. Pour the cream into the chilled bowl, and beat until soft peaks form, 1 to 3 minutes, depending on the freshness of your cream.
5. Take the chilled yogurt mixture out of the refrigerator. Gently fold it into the whipped cream using a rubber scraper; lift and turn the mixture to prevent the cream from deflating. Chill until serving, at least 15 minutes but no longer than 1 hour.
6. To serve, spoon the lemon fool into four glasses or dessert dishes and drizzle with the remaining ½ tablespoon of honey. Top with fresh fruit and mint, if desired.

Per Serving
calories: 171 | fat: 9g | protein: 3g
carbs: 20g | fiber: 0g | sodium: 37mg

Nut Butter Cup

Prep time: 10 minutes | Cook time: 0 minutes | Serves 8

½ cup crunchy almond butter (no sugar added)
½ cup light fruity extra-virgin olive oil
¼ cup ground flaxseed
2 tablespoons unsweetened cocoa
powder
1 teaspoon vanilla extract
1 teaspoon ground cinnamon (optional)
1 to 2 teaspoons sugar-free sweetener of choice (optional)

1. In a mixing bowl, combine the almond butter, olive oil, flaxseed, cocoa powder, vanilla, cinnamon (if using), and sweetener (if using) and stir well with a spatula to combine. Mixture will be a thick liquid.
2. Pour into 8 mini muffin liners and freeze until solid, at least 12 hours. Store in the freezer to maintain their shape.

Per Serving (1 fat bomb)
calories: 240 | fat: 23g | protein: 3g
carbs: 5g | fiber: 2g | sodium: 3mg

Dark Chocolate and Avocado Mousse

Prep time: 5 minutes | Cook time: 5 minutes | Serves 4 to 6

8 ounces (227 g) dark chocolate (60% cocoa or higher), chopped
¼ cup unsweetened coconut milk
2 tablespoons coconut oil
2 ripe avocados, deseeded
¼ cup raw honey
Sea salt, to taste

1. Put the chocolate in a saucepan. Pour in the coconut milk and add the coconut oil.
2. Cook for 3 minutes or until the chocolate and coconut oil melt. Stir constantly.
3. Put the avocado in a food processor, then drizzle with honey and melted chocolate. Pulse to combine until smooth.
4. Pour the mixture in a serving bowl, then sprinkle with salt. Refrigerate to chill for 30 minutes and serve.

Per Serving
calories: 654 | fat: 46g | protein: 7g
carbs: 55g | fiber: 9g | sodium: 112mg

Flourless Brownies with Balsamic Raspberry Sauce

Prep time: 10 minutes | Cook time: 30 minutes | Serves 2

For the Raspberry Sauce:

¼ cup good-quality balsamic vinegar
1 cup frozen raspberries
For the Brownie:
½ cup black beans with no added salt, rinsed
1 large egg
1 tablespoon olive oil
½ teaspoon vanilla extract
4 tablespoons unsweetened cocoa powder
¼ cup sugar
¼ teaspoon baking powder
Pinch salt
¼ cup dark chocolate chips

Make the Raspberry Sauce

1. Combine the balsamic vinegar and raspberries in a saucepan and bring the mixture to a boil. Reduce the heat to medium and let the sauce simmer for 15 minutes, or until reduced to ½ cup. If desired, strain the seeds and set the sauce aside until the brownie is ready.

Make the Brownie

2. Preheat the oven to 350ºF (180ºC) and set the rack to the middle position. Grease two 8-ounce ramekins and place them on a baking sheet.
3. In a food processor, combine the black beans, egg, olive oil, and vanilla. Purée the mixture for 1 to 2 minutes, or until it's smooth and the beans are completely broken down. Scrape down the sides of the bowl a few times to make sure everything is well-incorporated.
4. Add the cocoa powder, sugar, baking powder, and salt and purée again to combine the dry ingredients, scraping down the sides of the bowl as needed.
5. Stir the chocolate chips into the batter by hand. Reserve a few if you like, to sprinkle over the top of the brownies when they come out of the oven.
6. Pour the brownies into the prepared ramekins and bake for 15 minutes, or until firm. The center will look slightly undercooked. If you prefer a firmer brownie, leave it in the oven for another 5 minutes, or until a toothpick inserted in the middle comes out clean.
7. Remove the brownies from the oven. If desired, sprinkle any remaining chocolate chips over the top and let them melt into the warm brownies.
8. Let the brownies cool for a few minutes and top with warm raspberry sauce to serve.

Per Serving
calories: 447 | fat: 15g | protein: 10g
carbs: 68g | fiber: 13g | sodium: 124mg

Fruit and Nut Dark Chocolate Bark

Prep time: 15 minutes | Cook time: 5 minutes | Serves 2

2 tablespoons chopped nuts (almonds, pecans, walnuts, hazelnuts, pistachios, or any combination of those)
3 ounces (85 g) good-quality dark chocolate chips (about ⅔ cup)
¼ cup chopped dried fruit (apricots, blueberries, figs, prunes, or any combination of those)

1. Line a sheet pan with parchment paper.
2. Place the nuts in a skillet over medium-high heat and toast them for 60 seconds, or just until they're fragrant.
3. Place the chocolate in a microwave-safe glass bowl or measuring cup and microwave on high for 1 minute. Stir the chocolate and allow any unmelted chips to warm and melt. If necessary, heat for another 20 to 30 seconds, but keep a close eye on it to make sure it doesn't burn.
4. Pour the chocolate onto the sheet pan. Sprinkle the dried fruit and nuts over the chocolate evenly and gently pat in so they stick.
5. Transfer the sheet pan to the refrigerator for at least 1 hour to let the chocolate harden.
6. When solid, break into pieces. Store any leftover chocolate in the refrigerator or freezer.

Per Serving
calories: 284 | fat: 16g | protein: 4g
carbs: 39g | fiber: 2g | sodium: 2mg

Chocolate Dessert Hummus

Prep time: 15 minutes | Cook time: 0 minutes | Serves 2

Caramel:

2 tablespoons coconut oil
1 tablespoon maple syrup
1 tablespoon almond butter
Pinch salt

Hummus:

½ cup chickpeas, drained and rinsed
2 tablespoons unsweetened cocoa powder
1 tablespoon maple syrup, plus more to
taste
2 tablespoons almond milk, or more as needed, to thin
Pinch salt
2 tablespoons pecans

Make the Caramel

1. To make the caramel, put the coconut oil in a small microwave-safe bowl. If it's solid, microwave it for about 15 seconds to melt it.
2. Stir in the maple syrup, almond butter, and salt.
3. Place the caramel in the refrigerator for 5 to 10 minutes to thicken.

Make the Hummus

1. In a food processor, combine the chickpeas, cocoa powder, maple syrup, almond milk, and pinch of salt, and process until smooth. Scrape down the sides to make sure everything is incorporated.
2. If the hummus seems too thick, add another tablespoon of almond milk.
3. Add the pecans and pulse 6 times to roughly chop them.
4. Transfer the hummus to a serving bowl and when the caramel is thickened, swirl it into the hummus. Gently fold it in, but don't mix it in completely.
5. Serve with fresh fruit or pretzels.

Per Serving

calories: 321 | fat: 22g | protein: 7g
carbs: 30g | fiber: 6g | sodium: 100mg

Blackberry Lemon Panna Cotta

Prep time: 20 minutes | Cook time: 10 minutes | Serves 2

¾ cup half-and-half, divided
1 teaspoon unflavored powdered gelatin
½ cup heavy cream
3 tablespoons sugar
1 teaspoon lemon zest
1 tablespoon freshly squeezed lemon juice
1 teaspoon lemon extract
½ cup fresh blackberries
Lemon peels to garnish (optional)

1. Place ¼ cup of half-and-half in a small bowl.
2. Sprinkle the gelatin powder evenly over the half-and-half and set it aside for 10 minutes to hydrate.
3. In a saucepan, combine the remaining ½ cup of half-and-half, the heavy cream, sugar, lemon zest, lemon juice, and lemon extract. Heat the mixture over medium heat for 4 minutes, or until it's barely simmering—don't let it come to a full boil. Remove from the heat.
4. When the gelatin is hydrated (it will look like applesauce), add it into the warm cream mixture, whisking as the gelatin melts.
5. If there are any remaining clumps of gelatin, strain the liquid or remove the lumps with a spoon.
6. Pour the mixture into 2 dessert glasses or stemless wineglasses and refrigerate for at least 6 hours, or up to overnight.
7. Serve with the fresh berries and garnish with some strips of fresh lemon peel, if desired.

Per Serving

calories: 422 | fat: 33g | protein: 6g
carbs: 28g | fiber: 2g | sodium: 64mg

Pecan and Carrot Coconut Cake

Prep time: 10 minutes | Cook time: 45 minutes | Serves 12

½ cup coconut oil, at room temperature, plus more for greasing the baking dish
2 teaspoons pure vanilla extract
¼ cup pure maple syrup
6 eggs
½ cup coconut flour
1 teaspoon baking powder
1 teaspoon baking soda
½ teaspoon ground nutmeg
1 teaspoon ground cinnamon
⅛ teaspoon sea salt
½ cup chopped pecans
3 cups finely grated carrots

1. Preheat the oven to 350ºF (180ºC). Grease a 13-by-9-inch baking dish with coconut oil.
2. Combine the vanilla extract, maple syrup, and ½ cup of coconut oil in a large bowl. Stir to mix well.
3. Break the eggs in the bowl and whisk to combine well. Set aside.
4. Combine the coconut flour, baking powder, baking soda, nutmeg, cinnamon, and salt in a separate bowl. Stir to mix well.
5. Make a well in the center of the flour mixture, then pour the egg mixture into the well. Stir to combine well.
6. Add the pecans and carrots to the bowl and toss to mix well. Pour the mixture in the single layer on the baking dish.
7. Bake in the preheated oven for 45 minutes or until puffed and the cake spring back when lightly press with your fingers.
8. Remove the cake from the oven. Allow to cool for at least 15 minutes, then serve.

Per Serving
calories: 255 | fat: 21g | protein: 5g
carbs: 12g | fiber: 2g | sodium: 202mg

Baklava with Syrup

Prep time: 10 minutes | Cook time: 30 minutes | Serves 12

1½ cups finely chopped walnuts
1 teaspoon ground cinnamon
¼ teaspoon ground cardamom (optional)
1 cup water
½ cup sugar
½ cup honey
2 tablespoons freshly squeezed lemon juice
1 cup salted butter, melted (optional)
20 large sheets phyllo pastry dough, at room temperature

1. Preheat the oven to 350ºF (180ºC).
2. In a small bowl, gently mix the walnuts, cinnamon, and cardamom (if using) and set aside.
3. In a small pot, bring the water, sugar, honey, and lemon juice just to a boil. Remove from the heat.
4. Put the butter in a small bowl. Onto an ungreased 9-by-13-inch baking sheet, put 1 layer of phyllo dough and slowly brush with butter. Be careful not to tear the phyllo sheets as you butter them. Carefully layer 1 or 2 more phyllo sheets, brushing each with butter in the baking pan, and then layer ⅛ of the nut mix; layer 2 sheets and add another ⅛ of the nut mix; repeat with 2 sheets and nuts until you run out of nuts and dough, topping with the remaining phyllo dough sheets.
5. Slice 4 lines into the baklava lengthwise and make another 4 or 5 slices diagonally across the pan.
6. Put in the oven and cook for 30 to 40 minutes, or until golden brown.
7. Remove the baklava from the oven and immediately cover it with the syrup.

Per Serving
calories: 443 | fat: 26g | protein: 6g
carbs: 47g | fiber: 3g | sodium: 344mg

Baked Lemon Cookies

Prep time: 10 minutes | Cook time: 10 minutes | Makes 12 cookies

Nonstick cooking spray
¾ cup granulated sugar
½ cup butter (optional)
1½ teaspoons vinegar
1 large egg
1 teaspoon grated lemon zest
1¾ cups flour
1 teaspoon baking powder
¼ teaspoon baking soda
¾ cup confectioners' sugar
¼ cup freshly squeezed lemon juice
1 teaspoon finely grated lemon zest

1. Preheat the oven to 350ºF (180ºC). Spray a baking sheet with cooking spray and set aside.
2. In a medium bowl, cream the sugar and butter (if desired). Next, stir in the vinegar, and then add the egg and lemon zest, and mix well. Sift the flour, baking powder, and baking soda into the bowl and mix until combined.
3. Spoon the mixture onto a prepared baking sheet in 12 equal heaps. Bake for 10 to 12 minutes. Be sure not to burn the bottoms.
4. While the cookies are baking, make the lemon glaze in a small bowl by mixing the sugar, lemon juice, and lemon zest together.
5. Remove the cookies from the oven and brush with lemon glaze.

Per Serving
calories: 233 | fat: 8g | protein: 2g
carbs: 39g | fiber: 1g | sodium:132 mg

Chilled Fruit Kebabs with Dark Chocolate

Prep time: 5 minutes | Cook time: 1 minute | Serves 6

12 strawberries, hulled
12 cherries, pitted
24 seedless red or
green grapes
24 blueberries
8 ounces (227 g) dark chocolate

1. Line a large, rimmed baking sheet with parchment paper. On your work surface, lay out six 12-inch wooden skewers.
2. Thread the fruit onto the skewers, following this pattern: 1 strawberry, 1 cherry, 2 grapes, 2 blueberries, 1 strawberry, 1 cherry, 2 grapes, and 2 blueberries (or vary according to taste!). Place the kebabs on the prepared baking sheet.
3. In a medium, microwave-safe bowl, heat the chocolate in the microwave for 1 minute on high. Stir until the chocolate is completely melted.
4. Spoon the melted chocolate into a small plastic sandwich bag. Twist the bag closed right above the chocolate, and snip the corner of the bag off with scissors. Squeeze the bag to drizzle lines of chocolate over the kebabs.
5. Place the sheet in the freezer and chill for 20 minutes before serving.

Per Serving
calories: 297 | fat: 16g | protein: 4g
carbs: 35g | fiber: 5g | sodium: 12mg

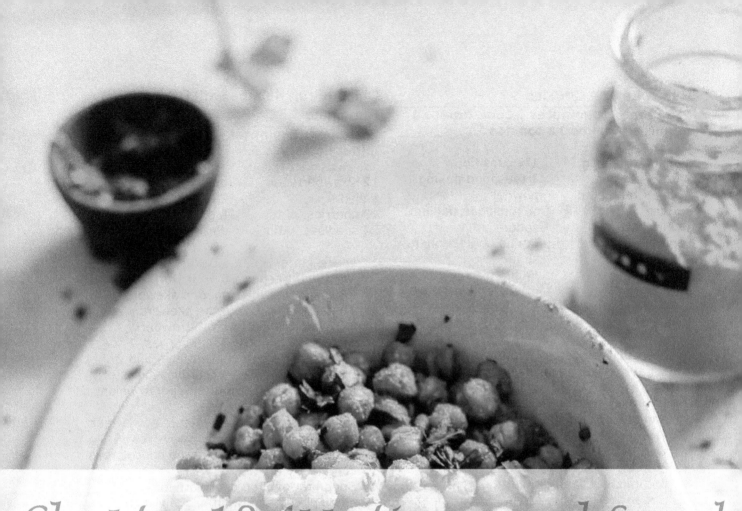
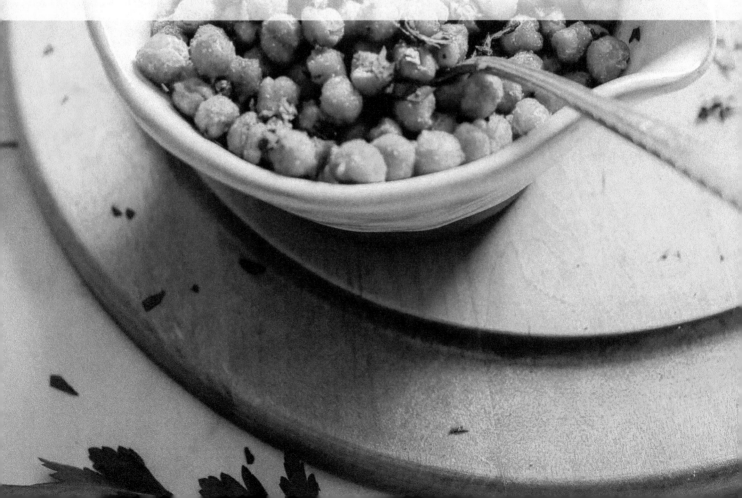

Chapter 18 Appetizers and Snacks

Citrus Garlic Marinated Olives

Prep time: 10 minutes | Cook time: 0 minutes | Makes 2 cups

2 cups mixed green olives with pits
¼ cup red wine vinegar
¼ cup extra-virgin olive oil
4 garlic cloves, finely minced
Zest and juice of
2 clementines or 1 large orange
1 teaspoon red pepper flakes
2 bay leaves
½ teaspoon ground cumin
½ teaspoon ground allspice

1. In a large glass bowl or jar, combine the olives, vinegar, oil, garlic, orange zest and juice, red pepper flakes, bay leaves, cumin, and allspice and mix well. Cover and refrigerate for at least 4 hours or up to a week to allow the olives to marinate, tossing again before serving.

Per Serving (¼ cup)
calories: 133 | fat: 14g | protein: 1g
carbs: 3g | fiber: 2g | sodium: 501mg

Crunchy Chili Chickpeas

Prep time: 5 minutes | Cook time: 15 minutes | Serves 4

1 (15-ounce / 425-g) can cooked chickpeas, drained and rinsed
1 tablespoon olive oil
¼ teaspoon salt
⅛ teaspoon chili powder
⅛ teaspoon garlic powder
⅛ teaspoon paprika

1. Preheat the air fryer to 380ºF (193ºC).
2. In a medium bowl, toss all of the ingredients together until the chickpeas are well coated.
3. Pour the chickpeas into the air fryer and spread them out in a single layer.
4. Roast for 15 minutes, stirring once halfway through the cook time.

Per Serving
calories: 109 | fat: 5g | protein: 4g
carbs: 13g | fiber: 4g | sodium: 283mg

Falafel Balls with Garlic-Yogurt Sauce

Prep time: 5 minutes | Cook time: 15 minutes | Serves 4

Falafel:
1 (15-ounce / 425-g) can chickpeas, drained and rinsed
½ cup fresh parsley
2 garlic cloves, minced
½ tablespoon ground cumin
1 tablespoon whole wheat flour
Salt, to taste

Garlic-Yogurt Sauce:
1 cup nonfat plain Greek yogurt
1 garlic clove, minced
1 tablespoon chopped
fresh dill
2 tablespoons lemon juice

Make the Falafel
1. Preheat the air fryer to 360ºF (182ºC).
2. Put the chickpeas into a food processor. Pulse until mostly chopped, then add the parsley, garlic, and cumin and pulse for another 1 to 2 minutes, or until the ingredients are combined and turning into a dough.
3. Add the flour. Pulse a few more times until combined. The dough will have texture, but the chickpeas should be pulsed into small bits.
4. Using clean hands, roll the dough into 8 balls of equal size, then pat the balls down a bit so they are about ½-thick disks.
5. Spray the basket of the air fryer with olive oil cooking spray, then place the falafel patties in the basket in a single layer, making sure they don't touch each other.
6. Fry in the air fryer for 15 minutes.

Make the Garlic-Yogurt Sauce
7. In a small bowl, combine the yogurt, garlic, dill, and lemon juice.
8. Once the falafel are done cooking and nicely browned on all sides, remove them from the air fryer and season with salt.
9. Serve hot with a side of dipping sauce.

Per Serving
calories: 151 | fat: 2g | protein: 12g
carbs: 22g | fiber: 5g | sodium: 141mg

Mediterranean White Beans with Basil

Prep time: 2 minutes | Cook time: 19 minutes | Serves 2

1 (15-ounce / 425-g) can cooked white beans
2 tablespoons olive oil
1 teaspoon fresh sage, chopped

¼ teaspoon garlic powder
¼ teaspoon salt, divided
1 teaspoon chopped fresh basil

1. Preheat the air fryer to 380ºF (193ºC).
2. In a medium bowl, mix together the beans, olive oil, sage, garlic, ⅛ teaspoon salt, and basil.
3. Pour the white beans into the air fryer and spread them out in a single layer.
4. Bake for 10 minutes. Stir and continue cooking for an additional 5 to 9 minutes, or until they reach your preferred level of crispiness.
5. Toss with the remaining ⅛ teaspoon salt before serving.

Per Serving

calories: 308 | fat: 14g | protein: 13g
carbs: 34g | fiber: 9g | sodium: 294mg

Beet Chips

Prep time: 10 minutes | Cook time: 30 minutes | Serves 6

4 medium beets, rinse and thinly sliced
1 teaspoon sea salt

2 tablespoons olive oil
Hummus, for serving

1. Preheat the air fryer to 380ºF (193ºC).
2. In a large bowl, toss the beets with sea salt and olive oil until well coated.
3. Put the beet slices into the air fryer and spread them out in a single layer.
4. Fry for 10 minutes. Stir, then fry for an additional 10 minutes. Stir again, then fry for a final 5 to 10 minutes, or until the chips reach the desired crispiness.
5. Serve with a favorite hummus.

Per Serving

calories: 63 | fat: 5g | protein: 1g
carbs: 5g | fiber: 2g | sodium: 430mg

Healthy Deviled Eggs with Greek Yogurt

Prep time: 15 minutes | Cook time: 15 minutes | Serves 4

4 eggs
¼ cup nonfat plain Greek yogurt
1 teaspoon chopped fresh dill
⅛ teaspoon salt

⅛ teaspoon paprika
⅛ teaspoon garlic powder
Chopped fresh parsley, for garnish

1. Preheat the air fryer to 270ºF (132ºC).
2. Place the eggs in a single layer in the air fryer basket and cook for 15 minutes.
3. Quickly remove the eggs from the air fryer and place them into a cold water bath. Let the eggs cool in the water for 10 minutes before removing and peeling them.
4. After peeling the eggs, cut them in half.
5. Spoon the yolk into a small bowl. Add the yogurt, dill, salt, paprika, and garlic powder and mix until smooth.
6. Spoon or pipe the yolk mixture into the halved egg whites. Serve with a sprinkle of fresh parsley on top.

Per Serving

calories: 80 | fat: 5g | protein: 8g
carbs: 1g | fiber: 0g | sodium: 149mg

Spiced Cashews

Prep time: 5 minutes | Cook time: 10 minutes | Serves 4

2 cups raw cashews
2 tablespoons olive oil
¼ teaspoon salt
¼ teaspoon chili

powder
⅛ teaspoon garlic powder
⅛ teaspoon smoked paprika

1. Preheat the air fryer to 360ºF (182ºC).
2. In a large bowl, toss all of the ingredients together.
3. Pour the cashews into the air fryer basket and roast them for 5 minutes. Shake the basket, then cook for 5 minutes more.
4. Serve immediately.

Per Serving

calories: 476 | fat: 40g | protein: 14g
carbs: 23g | fiber: 3g | sodium: 151mg

Sweet Potato Chips

Prep time: 5 minutes | Cook time: 15 minutes | Serves 2

1 large sweet potato, thinly sliced
⅛ teaspoon salt
2 tablespoons olive oil

1. Preheat the air fryer to 380ºF (193ºC).
2. In a small bowl, toss the sweet potatoes, salt, and olive oil together until the potatoes are well coated.
3. Put the sweet potato slices into the air fryer and spread them out in a single layer.
4. Fry for 10 minutes. Stir, then air fry for 3 to 5 minutes more, or until the chips reach the preferred level of crispiness.

Per Serving
calories: 175 | fat: 14g | protein: 1g
carbs: 13g | fiber: 2g | sodium: 191mg

Cranberry Chocolate Granola Bars

Prep time: 5 minutes | Cook time: 15 minutes | Serves 6

2 cups certified gluten-free quick oats
2 tablespoons sugar-free dark chocolate chunks
2 tablespoons unsweetened dried cranberries
3 tablespoons unsweetened shredded coconut
½ cup raw honey
1 teaspoon ground cinnamon
⅛ teaspoon salt
2 tablespoons olive oil

1. Preheat the air fryer to 360ºF (182ºC). Line an 8-by-8-inch baking dish with parchment paper that comes up the side so you can lift it out after cooking.
2. In a large bowl, mix together all of the ingredients until well combined.
3. Press the oat mixture into the pan in an even layer.
4. Place the pan into the air fryer basket and bake for 15 minutes.
5. Remove the pan from the air fryer, and lift the granola cake out of the pan using the edges of the parchment paper.
6. Allow to cool for 5 minutes before slicing into 6 equal bars.

7. Serve immediately, or wrap in plastic wrap and store at room temperature for up to 1 week.

Per Serving
calories: 272 | fat: 10g | protein: 6g
carbs: 55g | fiber: 5g | sodium: 74mg

Carrot Cake Cupcakes with Walnuts

Prep time: 10 minutes | Cook time: 12 minutes | Serves 6

Olive oil cooking spray
1 cup grated carrots
¼ cup raw honey
¼ cup olive oil
½ teaspoon vanilla extract
1 egg
¼ cup unsweetened applesauce
1 ⅓ cups whole wheat flour
¾ teaspoon baking powder
½ teaspoon baking soda
½ teaspoon ground cinnamon
¼ teaspoon ground nutmeg
⅛ teaspoon ground ginger
⅛ teaspoon salt
¼ cup chopped walnuts
2 tablespoons chopped golden raisins

1. Preheat the air fryer to 380ºF (193ºC). Lightly coat the inside of six silicone muffin cups or a six-cup muffin tin with olive oil cooking spray.
2. In a medium bowl, mix together the carrots, honey, olive oil, vanilla extract, egg, and unsweetened applesauce.
3. In a separate medium bowl, whisk together the flour, baking powder, baking soda, cinnamon, nutmeg, ginger, and salt.
4. Add the wet ingredients to the dry ingredients, mixing until just combined.
5. Gently fold in the walnuts and raisins. Fill the muffin cups or tin three-quarters full with the batter, and place them in the air fryer basket.
6. Bake for 10 to 12 minutes, or until a toothpick inserted in the center of a cupcake comes out clean.
7. Serve immediately or store in an airtight container until ready to serve.

Per Serving
calories: 277 | fat: 14g | protein: 6g
carbs: 36g | fiber: 4g | sodium: 182mg

Roasted Figs with Goat Cheese

Prep time: 5 minutes | Cook time: 10 minutes | Serves 4

8 fresh figs
2 ounces (57 g) goat cheese
¼ teaspoon ground

cinnamon
1 tablespoon honey, plus more for serving
1 tablespoon olive oil

1. Preheat the air fryer to 360ºF (182ºC).
2. Cut the stem off of each fig.
3. Cut an X into the top of each fig, cutting halfway down the fig. Leave the base intact.
4. In a small bowl, mix together the goat cheese, cinnamon, and honey.
5. Spoon the goat cheese mixture into the cavity of each fig.
6. Place the figs in a single layer in the air fryer basket. Drizzle the olive oil over top of the figs and roast for 10 minutes.
7. Serve with an additional drizzle of honey.

Per Serving
calories: 158 | fat: 7g | protein: 3g
carbs: 24g | fiber: 3g | sodium: 61mg

Homemade Trail Mix

Prep time: 10 minutes | Cook time: 10 minutes | Makes 4 cups

1 tablespoon olive oil
1 tablespoon maple syrup
1 teaspoon vanilla
½ teaspoon cardamom
½ teaspoon allspice
2 cups mixed, unsalted nuts

¼ cup unsalted pumpkin or sunflower seeds
½ cup dried apricots, diced or thinly sliced
½ cup dried figs, diced or thinly sliced
Pinch salt

1. Combine the olive oil, maple syrup, vanilla, cardamom, and allspice in a large sauté pan over medium heat. Stir to combine.
2. Add the nuts and seeds and stir well to coat. Let the nuts and seeds toast for about 10 minutes, stirring frequently.
3. Remove from the heat, and add the dried apricots and figs. Stir everything well and season with salt.
4. Store in an airtight container.

Per Serving (½ cup)
calories: 261 | fat: 18g | protein: 6g
carbs: 23g | fiber: 5g | sodium: 26mg

Spiced Roasted Chickpeas

Prep time: 15 minutes | Cook time: 35 minutes | Serves 2

Seasoning Mix:
¾ teaspoon cumin
½ teaspoon coriander
½ teaspoon salt
¼ teaspoon freshly ground black pepper
¼ teaspoon paprika

¼ teaspoon cardamom
¼ teaspoon cinnamon
¼ teaspoon allspice

Chickpeas:
1 (15-ounce / 425-g) can chickpeas, drained and rinsed

1 tablespoon olive oil
¼ teaspoon salt

Make the Seasoning Mix
1. In a small bowl, combine the cumin, coriander, salt, freshly ground black pepper, paprika, cardamom, cinnamon, and allspice. Stir well to combine and set aside.

Make the Chickpeas
1. Preheat the oven to 400ºF (205ºC) and set the rack to the middle position. Line a baking sheet with parchment paper.
2. Pat the rinsed chickpeas with paper towels or roll them in a clean kitchen towel to dry off any water.
3. Place the chickpeas in a bowl and season them with the olive oil and salt.
4. Add the chickpeas to the lined baking sheet (reserve the bowl) and roast them for about 25 to 35 minutes, turning them over once or twice while cooking. Most should be light brown. Taste one or two to make sure they are slightly crisp.
5. Place the roasted chickpeas back into the bowl and sprinkle them with the seasoning mix. Toss lightly to combine. Taste, and add additional salt if needed. Serve warm.

Per Serving
calories: 268 | fat: 11g | protein: 11g
carbs: 35g | fiber: 10g | sodium: 301mg

Citrus-Thyme Chickpeas

Prep time: 5 minutes | Cook time: 23 minutes | Serves 4

1 (15-ounce / 425-g) can chickpeas, drained and rinsed	chopped fresh thyme leaves
2 teaspoons extra-virgin olive oil	⅛ teaspoon kosher or sea salt
¼ teaspoon dried thyme or ½ teaspoon	½ teaspoon zest of ½ orange

1. Preheat the oven to 450ºF (235ºC).
2. Spread the chickpeas on a clean kitchen towel, and rub gently until dry.
3. Spread the chickpeas on a large, rimmed baking sheet. Drizzle with the oil, and sprinkle with the thyme and salt. Using a Microplane or citrus zester, zest about half of the orange over the chickpeas. Mix well using your hands.
4. Bake for 10 minutes, then open the oven door and, using an oven mitt, give the baking sheet a quick shake. (Do not remove the sheet from the oven.) Bake for 10 minutes more. Taste the chickpeas (carefully!). If they are golden but you think they could be a bit crunchier, bake for 3 minutes more before serving.

Per Serving
calories: 97 | fat: 2g | protein: 5g
carbs: 14g | fiber: 4g | sodium: 232mg

Crispy Seedy Crackers

Prep time: 10 minutes | Cook time: 10 minutes | Makes 24 crackers

1 cup almond flour	soda
1 tablespoon sesame seeds	¼ teaspoon salt
1 tablespoon flaxseed	Freshly ground black pepper, to taste
1 tablespoon chia seeds	1 large egg, at room temperature
¼ teaspoon baking	

1. Preheat the oven to 350ºF (180ºC).
2. In a large bowl, combine the almond flour, sesame seeds, flaxseed, chia seeds, baking soda, salt, and pepper and stir well.
3. In a small bowl, whisk the egg until well beaten. Add to the dry ingredients and stir well to combine and form the dough into a ball.
4. Place one layer of parchment paper on your counter-top and place the dough on top. Cover with a second layer of parchment and, using a rolling pin, roll the dough to ⅛-inch thickness, aiming for a rectangular shape.
5. Cut the dough into 1- to 2-inch crackers and bake on parchment until crispy and slightly golden, 10 to 15 minutes, depending on thickness. Alternatively, you can bake the large rolled dough prior to cutting and break into free-form crackers once baked and crispy.
6. Store in an airtight container in the fridge for up to 1 week.

Per Serving (6 crackers)
calories: 119 | fat: 8g | protein: 5g
carbs: 4g | fiber: 2g | sodium: 242mg

Mediterranean Nutty Fat Bombs

Prep time: 5 minutes | Cook time: 0 minutes | Makes 6 fat bombs

1 cup crumbled goat cheese	olives, finely chopped
4 tablespoons jarred pesto	½ cup finely chopped walnuts
12 pitted Kalamata	1 tablespoon chopped fresh rosemary

1. In a medium bowl, combine the goat cheese, pesto, and olives and mix well using a fork. Place in the refrigerator for at least 4 hours to harden.
2. Using your hands, form the mixture into 6 balls, about ¾-inch diameter. The mixture will be sticky.
3. In a small bowl, place the walnuts and rosemary and roll the goat cheese balls in the nut mixture to coat.
4. Store the fat bombs in the refrigerator for up to 1 week or in the freezer for up to 1 month.

Per Serving (1 fat bomb)
calories: 166 | fat: 14g | protein: 5g
carbs: 4g | fiber: 1g | sodium: 337mg

Fried Halloumi with Tomato

Prep time: 2 minutes | Cook time: 5 minutes | Serves 2

3 ounces (85 g) Halloumi cheese, cut crosswise into 2 thinner, rectangular pieces
2 teaspoons prepared

pesto sauce, plus additional for drizzling
1 medium tomato, sliced

1. Heat a nonstick skillet over medium-high heat and place the slices of Halloumi in the hot pan. After about 2 minutes, check to see if the cheese is golden on the bottom. If it is, flip the slices, top each with 1 teaspoon of pesto, and cook for another 2 minutes, or until the second side is golden.
2. Serve with slices of tomato and a drizzle of pesto, if desired, on the side.

Per Serving
calories: 177 | fat: 14g | protein: 10g
carbs: 4g | fiber: 1g | sodium: 233mg

Cucumber Cup Appetizers

Prep time: 5 minutes | Cook time: 0 minutes | Serves 2

1 medium cucumber (about 8 ounces / 227 g, 8 to 9 inches long)
½ cup hummus (any flavor) or white bean

dip
4 or 5 cherry tomatoes, sliced in half
2 tablespoons fresh basil, minced

1. Slice the ends off the cucumber (about ½ inch from each side) and slice the cucumber into 1-inch pieces.
2. With a paring knife or a spoon, scoop most of the seeds from the inside of each cucumber piece to make a cup, being careful to not cut all the way through.
3. Fill each cucumber cup with about 1 tablespoon of hummus or bean dip.
4. Top each with a cherry tomato half and a sprinkle of fresh minced basil.

Per Serving
calories: 135 | fat: 6g | protein: 6g
carbs: 16g | fiber: 5g | sodium: 242mg

Rosemary and Honey Almonds

Prep time: 5 minutes | Cook time: 10 minutes | Serves 6

1 cup raw, whole, shelled almonds
1 tablespoon minced fresh rosemary
¼ teaspoon kosher

or sea salt
1 tablespoon honey
Nonstick cooking spray

1. In a large skillet over medium heat, combine the almonds, rosemary, and salt. Stir frequently for 1 minute.
2. Drizzle in the honey and cook for another 3 to 4 minutes, stirring frequently, until the almonds are coated and just starting to darken around the edges.
3. Remove from the heat. Using a spatula, spread the almonds onto a pan coated with nonstick cooking spray. Cool for 10 minutes or so. Break up the almonds before serving.

Per Serving
calories: 13 | fat: 1g | protein: 1g
carbs: 3g | fiber: 1g | sodium: 97mg

Balsamic Artichoke Antipasto

Prep time: 5 minutes | Cook time: 0 minutes | Serves 4

1 (12-ounce / 340-g) jar roasted red peppers, drained, stemmed, and seeded
8 artichoke hearts, either frozen (thawed), or jarred (drained)

1 (16-ounce / 454-g) can garbanzo beans, drained
1 cup whole Kalamata olives, drained
¼ cup balsamic vinegar
½ teaspoon salt

1. Cut the peppers into ½-inch slices and put them into a large bowl.
2. Cut the artichoke hearts into quarters, and add them to the bowl.
3. Add the garbanzo beans, olives, balsamic vinegar, and salt.
4. Toss all the ingredients together. Serve chilled.

Per Serving
calories: 281 | fat: 14g | protein: 7g
carbs: 30g | fiber: 9g | sodium: 1237mg

Pickled Turnips

Prep time: 5 minutes | Cook time: 0 minutes | Makes about 1 quart

1 pound (454 g) turnips, washed well, peeled, and cut into 1-inch batons
1 small beet, roasted, peeled, and cut into 1-inch batons
2 garlic cloves, smashed
1 teaspoon dried Turkish oregano
3 cups warm water
½ cup red wine vinegar
½ cup white vinegar

1. In a jar, combine the turnips, beet, garlic, and oregano. Pour the water and vinegars over the vegetables, cover, then shake well and put it in the refrigerator. The turnips will be pickled after 1 hour.

Per Serving (1 to 2 tablespoons)
calories: 8 | fat: 0g | protein: 1g
carbs: 1g | fiber: 0g | sodium: 6mg

Garlic and Herb Marinated Artichokes

Prep time: 10 minutes | Cook time: 0 minutes | Makes 2 cups

2 (13¾-ounce / 390-g) cans artichoke hearts, drained and quartered
¾ cup extra-virgin olive oil
4 small garlic cloves, crushed with the back of a knife
1 tablespoon fresh rosemary leaves
2 teaspoons chopped fresh oregano or 1 teaspoon dried oregano
1 teaspoon red pepper flakes (optional)
1 teaspoon salt

1. In a medium bowl, combine the artichoke hearts, olive oil, garlic, rosemary, oregano, red pepper flakes (if using), and salt. Toss to combine well.
2. Store in an airtight glass container in the refrigerator and marinate for at least 24 hours before using. Store in the refrigerator for up to 2 weeks.

Per Serving (¼ cup)
calories: 275 | fat: 27g | protein: 4g
carbs: 11g | fiber: 4g | sodium: 652mg

Turkish Spiced Mixed-Nuts

Prep time: 10 minutes | Cook time: 5 minutes | Serves 4 to 6

1 tablespoon extra-virgin olive oil
1 cup mixed nuts (walnuts, almonds, cashews, peanuts)
2 tablespoons paprika
1 tablespoon dried mint
½ tablespoon ground cinnamon
½ tablespoon kosher salt
¼ tablespoon garlic powder
¼ teaspoon freshly ground black pepper
⅛ tablespoon ground cumin

1. In a small to medium saucepan, heat the oil on low heat.
2. Once the oil is warm, add the nuts, paprika, mint, cinnamon, salt, garlic powder, pepper, and cumin and stir continually until the spices are well incorporated with the nuts.

Per Serving
calories: 204 | fat: 17g | protein: 6g
carbs: 10g | fiber: 3g | sodium: 874mg

Air-Fried Popcorn with Garlic Salt

Prep time: 5 minutes | Cook time: 8 minutes | Serves 2

2 tablespoons olive oil
¼ cup popcorn kernels
1 teaspoon garlic salt

1. Preheat the air fryer to 380ºF (193ºC).
2. Tear a square of aluminum foil the size of the bottom of the air fryer and place into the air fryer.
3. Drizzle olive oil over the top of the foil, and then pour in the popcorn kernels.
4. Roast for 8 to 10 minutes, or until the popcorn stops popping.
5. Transfer the popcorn to a large bowl and sprinkle with garlic salt before serving.

Per Serving
calories: 245 | fat: 14g | protein: 4g
carbs: 25g | fiber: 5g | sodium: 885mg

Apple Chips with Chocolate Tahini Sauce

Prep time: 10 minutes | Cook time: 0 minutes | Serves 2

2 tablespoons tahini
1 tablespoon maple syrup
1 tablespoon unsweetened cocoa powder
1 to 2 tablespoons

warm water (or more if needed)
2 medium apples
1 tablespoon roasted, salted sunflower seeds

1. In a small bowl, mix together the tahini, maple syrup, and cocoa powder. Add warm water, a little at a time, until thin enough to drizzle. Do not microwave it to thin it, it won't work.
2. Slice the apples crosswise into round slices, and then cut each piece in half to make a chip.
3. Lay the apple chips out on a plate and drizzle them with the chocolate tahini sauce.
4. Sprinkle sunflower seeds over the apple chips.

Per Serving
calories: 261 | fat: 11g | protein: 5g
carbs: 43g | fiber: 8g | sodium: 21mg

Mediterranean-Style Trail Mix

Prep time: 10 minutes | Cook time: 0 minutes | Serves 6

1 cup roughly chopped unsalted walnuts
½ cup roughly chopped salted almonds
½ cup shelled salted

pistachios
½ cup roughly chopped apricots
½ cup roughly chopped dates
⅓ cup dried figs, sliced in half

1. In a large zip-top bag, combine the walnuts, almonds, pistachios, apricots, dates, and figs and mix well.

Per Serving
calories: 348 | fat: 23g | protein: 9g
carbs: 33g | fiber: 6g | sodium: 95mg

Savory Mediterranean Spiced Popcorn

Prep time: 10 minutes | Cook time: 2 minutes | Serves 4 to 6

3 tablespoons extra-virgin olive oil
¼ teaspoon garlic powder
¼ teaspoon freshly ground black pepper
¼ teaspoon sea salt

⅛ teaspoon dried thyme
⅛ teaspoon dried oregano
12 cups plain popped popcorn

1. In a large sauté pan or skillet, heat the oil over medium heat, until shimmering, and then add the garlic powder, pepper, salt, thyme, and oregano until fragrant.
2. In a large bowl, drizzle the oil over the popcorn, toss, and serve.

Per Serving
calories: 183 | fat: 12g | protein: 3g
carbs: 19g | fiber: 3g | sodium: 146mg

Strawberry Caprese Skewers with Balsamic Glaze

Prep time: 15 minutes | Cook time: 10 minutes | Serves 2

½ cup balsamic vinegar
16 whole, hulled strawberries
12 small basil leaves

or 6 large leaves, halved
12 pieces of small Mozzarella balls

1. To make the balsamic glaze, pour the balsamic vinegar into a small saucepan and bring it to a boil. Reduce the heat to medium-low and simmer for 10 minutes, or until it's reduced by half and is thick enough to coat the back of a spoon.
2. On each of 4 wooden skewers, place a strawberry, a folded basil leaf, and a Mozzarella ball, repeating twice and adding a strawberry on the end. (Each skewer should have 4 strawberries, 3 basil leaves, and 3 Mozzarella balls.)
3. Drizzle 1 to 2 teaspoons of balsamic glaze over the skewers.

Per Serving
calories: 206 | fat: 10g | protein: 10g
carbs: 17g | fiber: 1g | sodium: 282mg

Lemon Marinated Feta and Artichokes

Prep time: 10 minutes | Cook time: 0 minutes | Makes 1½ cups

4 ounces (113 g) traditional Greek feta, cut into ½-inch cubes
4 ounces (113 g) drained artichoke hearts, quartered lengthwise
1/3 cup extra-virgin olive oil

Zest and juice of 1 lemon
2 tablespoons roughly chopped fresh rosemary
2 tablespoons roughly chopped fresh parsley
½ teaspoon black peppercorns

1. In a glass bowl or large glass jar, combine the feta and artichoke hearts. Add the olive oil, lemon zest and juice, rosemary, parsley, and peppercorns and toss gently to coat, being sure not to crumble the feta.
2. Cover and refrigerate for at least 4 hours, or up to 4 days. Pull out of the refrigerator 30 minutes before serving.

Per Serving (1/3 cup)
calories: 235 | fat: 23g | protein: 4g
carbs: 3g | fiber: 1g | sodium: 406mg

Salmon and Avocado Stuffed Cucumbers

Prep time: 10 minutes | Cook time: 0 minutes | Serves 4

2 large cucumbers, peeled
1 (4-ounce / 113-g) can red salmon
1 medium very ripe avocado, peeled, pitted, and mashed
1 tablespoon extra-virgin olive oil

Zest and juice of 1 lime
3 tablespoons chopped fresh cilantro
½ teaspoon salt
¼ teaspoon freshly ground black pepper

1. Slice the cucumber into 1-inch-thick segments and using a spoon, scrape seeds out of center of each segment and stand up on a plate.
2. In a medium bowl, combine the salmon, avocado, olive oil, lime zest and juice, cilantro, salt, and pepper and mix until creamy.

3. Spoon the salmon mixture into the center of each cucumber segment and serve chilled.

Per Serving
calories: 159 | fat: 11g | protein: 9g
carbs: 8g | fiber: 3g | sodium: 398mg

Fried Green Beans

Prep time: 5 minutes | Cook time: 5 minutes | Serves 4

Green Beans:
1 egg
2 tablespoons water
1 tablespoon whole wheat flour
¼ teaspoon paprika
½ teaspoon garlic

powder
½ teaspoon salt
¼ cup whole wheat bread crumbs
½ pound (227 g) whole green beans

Lemon-Yogurt Sauce:
½ cup nonfat plain Greek yogurt
1 tablespoon lemon juice

¼ teaspoon salt
⅛ teaspoon cayenne pepper

Make the Green Beans
1. Preheat the air fryer to 380°F (193°C).
2. In a medium shallow bowl, beat together the egg and water until frothy.
3. In a separate medium shallow bowl, whisk together the flour, paprika, garlic powder, and salt, then mix in the bread crumbs.
4. Spray the bottom of the air fryer with cooking spray.
5. Dip each green bean into the egg mixture, then into the bread crumb mixture, coating the outside with the crumbs. Place the green beans in a single layer in the bottom of the air fryer basket.
6. Fry in the air fryer for 5 minutes, or until the breading is golden brown.

Make the Lemon-Yogurt Sauce
1. In a small bowl, combine the yogurt, lemon juice, salt, and cayenne.
2. Serve the green bean fries alongside the lemon-yogurt sauce as a snack or appetizer.

Per Serving
calories: 88 | fat: 2g | protein: 7g
carbs: 12g | fiber: 2g | sodium: 502mg

Labneh Vegetable Parfaits

Prep time: 15 minutes | Cook time: 0 minutes | Serves 2

Labneh:

8 ounces (227 g) plain Greek yogurt (full-fat works best)
Generous pinch salt
1 teaspoon za'atar seasoning
1 teaspoon freshly squeezed lemon juice
Pinch lemon zest

Parfaits:

½ cup peeled, chopped cucumber
½ cup grated carrots
½ cup cherry tomatoes, halved

Make the Labneh

1. Line a strainer with cheesecloth and place it over a bowl.
2. Stir together the Greek yogurt and salt and place in the cheesecloth. Wrap it up and let it sit for 24 hours in the refrigerator.
3. When ready, unwrap the labneh and place it into a clean bowl. Stir in the za'atar, lemon juice, and lemon zest.

Make the Parfaits

1. Divide the cucumber between two clear glasses.
2. Top each portion of cucumber with about 3 tablespoons of labneh.
3. Divide the carrots between the glasses.
4. Top with another 3 tablespoons of the labneh.
5. Top parfaits with the cherry tomatoes.

Per Serving
calories: 143 | fat: 7g | protein: 5g
carbs: 16g | fiber: 2g | sodium: 187mg

Kalamata Olive Tapenade

Prep time: 10 minutes | Cook time: 0 minutes | Makes 2 cups

2 cups pitted Kalamata olives or other black olives
2 anchovy fillets, chopped
2 teaspoons chopped capers
1 garlic clove, finely minced
1 cooked egg yolk
1 teaspoon Dijon mustard
¼ cup extra-virgin olive oil
Vegetables, for serving (optional)

1. Rinse the olives in cold water and drain well.
2. In a food processor, blender, or a large jar (if using an immersion blender) place the drained olives, anchovies, capers, garlic, egg yolk, and Dijon. Process until it forms a thick paste.
3. With the food processor running, slowly stream in the olive oil.
4. Transfer to a small bowl, cover, and refrigerate at least 1 hour to let the flavors develop. Serve with your favorite crunchy vegetables.

Per Serving (¹/₃ cup)
calories: 179 | fat: 19g | protein: 2g
carbs: 3g | fiber: 2g | sodium: 812mg

Quinoa-Feta Stuffed Mushrooms

Prep time: 5 minutes | Cook time: 8 minutes | Serves 6

2 tablespoons finely diced red bell pepper
1 garlic clove, minced
¼ cup cooked quinoa
⅛ teaspoon salt
¼ teaspoon dried oregano
24 button mushrooms, stemmed
2 ounces (57 g) crumbled feta
3 tablespoons whole wheat bread crumbs
Olive oil cooking spray

1. Preheat the air fryer to 360ºF (182ºC).
2. In a small bowl, combine the bell pepper, garlic, quinoa, salt, and oregano.
3. Spoon the quinoa stuffing into the mushroom caps until just filled.
4. Add a small piece of feta to the top of each mushroom.
5. Sprinkle a pinch bread crumbs over the feta on each mushroom.
6. Spray the basket of the air fryer with olive oil cooking spray, then gently place the mushrooms into the basket, making sure that they don't touch each other. (Depending on the size of the air fryer, you may have to cook them in two batches.)
7. Place the basket into the air fryer and bake for 8 minutes.
8. Remove from the air fryer and serve.

Per Serving (4 mushrooms)
calories: 97 | fat: 4g | protein: 7g
carbs: 11g | fiber: 2g | sodium: 167mg

Caprese Stack with Burrata Cheese

Prep time: 5 minutes | Cook time: 0 minutes | Serves 4

1 large organic tomato, preferably heirloom
½ teaspoon salt
¼ teaspoon freshly ground black pepper
1 (4-ounce / 113-g) ball burrata cheese

8 fresh basil leaves, thinly sliced
2 tablespoons extra-virgin olive oil
1 tablespoon red wine or balsamic vinegar

1. Slice the tomato into 4 thick slices, removing any tough center core and sprinkle with salt and pepper. Place the tomatoes, seasoned-side up, on a plate.
2. On a separate rimmed plate, slice the burrata into 4 thick slices and place one slice on top of each tomato slice. Top each with one-quarter of the basil and pour any reserved burrata cream from the rimmed plate over top.
3. Drizzle with olive oil and vinegar and serve with a fork and knife.

Per Serving (1 stack)
calories: 153 | fat: 13g | protein: 7g
carbs: 2g | fiber: 1g | sodium: 469mg

Manchego Cheese Crackers

Prep time: 5 minutes | Cook time: 12 minutes | Makes 40 crackers

4 tablespoons butter, at room temperature (optional)
1 cup finely shredded Manchego cheese
1 cup almond flour

1 teaspoon salt, divided
¼ teaspoon freshly ground black pepper
1 large egg

1. Using an electric mixer, cream together the butter (if desired) and shredded cheese until well combined and smooth.
2. In a small bowl, combine the almond flour with ½ teaspoon salt and pepper. Slowly add the almond flour mixture to the cheese, mixing constantly until the dough just comes together to form a ball.
3. Transfer to a piece of parchment or plastic wrap and roll into a cylinder log about 1½ inches thick. Wrap tightly and refrigerate for at least 1 hour.

4. Preheat the oven to 350ºF (180ºC). Line two baking sheets with parchment paper or silicone baking mats.
5. To make the egg wash, in a small bowl, whisk together the egg and remaining ½ teaspoon salt.
6. Slice the refrigerated dough into small rounds, about ¼ inch thick, and place on the lined baking sheets.
7. Brush the tops of the crackers with egg wash and bake until the crackers are golden and crispy, 12 to 15 minutes. Remove from the oven and allow to cool on a wire rack.
8. Serve warm or, once fully cooled, store in an airtight container in the refrigerator for up to 1 week.

Per Serving (1 stack)
calories: 243 | fat: 22g | protein: 7g
carbs: 2g | fiber: 1g | sodium: 792mg

Mackerel Pâté with Horseradish

Prep time: 10 minutes | Cook time: 0 minutes | Serves 4

4 ounces (113 g) olive oil-packed wild-caught mackerel
2 ounces (57 g) goat cheese
Zest and juice of 1 lemon
2 tablespoons chopped fresh parsley
2 tablespoons chopped fresh

arugula
1 tablespoon extra-virgin olive oil
2 teaspoons chopped capers
1 to 2 teaspoons fresh horseradish (optional)
Crackers, cucumber rounds, endive spears, or celery, for serving (optional)

1. In a food processor, blender, or large bowl with immersion blender, combine the mackerel, goat cheese, lemon zest and juice, parsley, arugula, olive oil, capers, and horseradish (if using). Process or blend until smooth and creamy.
2. Serve with crackers, cucumber rounds, endive spears, or celery.
3. Store covered in the refrigerator for up to 1 week.

Per Serving
calories: 118 | fat: 8g | protein: 9g
carbs: 1g | fiber: 0g | sodium: 196mg

Whole Wheat Pita Chips

Prep time: 2 minutes | Cook time: 8 minutes | Serves 2

2 whole wheat pitas
1 tablespoon olive oil

½ teaspoon kosher salt

1. Preheat the air fryer to 360ºF (182ºC).
2. Cut each pita into 8 wedges.
3. In a medium bowl, toss the pita wedges, olive oil, and salt until the wedges are coated and the olive oil and salt are evenly distributed.
4. Place the pita wedges into the air fryer basket in an even layer and fry for 6 to 8 minutes. (The cooking time will vary depending upon how thick the pita is and how browned you prefer a chip.)
5. Season with additional salt, if desired. Serve alone or with a favorite dip.

Per Serving
calories: 230 | fat: 8g | protein: 6g
carbs: 35g | fiber: 4g | sodium: 706mg

Lemony Peanut Butter Hummus

Prep time: 10 minutes | Cook time: 0 minutes | Serves 6

1 (15-ounce / 425-g) can chickpeas, drained, liquid reserved
3 tablespoons freshly squeezed lemon juice (from about 1 large lemon)
2 tablespoons peanut butter

3 tablespoons extra-virgin olive oil, divided
2 garlic cloves
¼ teaspoon kosher or sea salt (optional)
Raw veggies or whole-grain crackers, for serving (optional)

1. In the bowl of a food processor, combine the chickpeas and 2 tablespoons of the reserved chickpea liquid with the lemon juice, peanut butter, 2 tablespoons of oil, and the garlic. Process the mixture for 1 minute. Scrape down the sides of the bowl with a rubber spatula. Process for 1 more minute, or until smooth.
2. Put in a serving bowl, drizzle with the remaining 1 tablespoon of olive oil, sprinkle with the salt, if using, and serve with veggies or crackers, if desired.

Per Serving
calories: 125 | fat: 5g | protein: 4g
carbs: 14g | fiber: 2g | sodium: 369mg

Greek-Style Potato Skins

Prep time: 5 minutes | Cook time: 45 minutes | Serves 4

2 russet potatoes
3 tablespoons olive oil, divided, plus more for drizzling (optional)
1 teaspoon kosher salt, divided
¼ teaspoon black pepper

2 tablespoons fresh cilantro, chopped, plus more for serving
¼ cup Kalamata olives, diced
¼ cup crumbled feta
Chopped fresh parsley, for garnish (optional)

1. Preheat the air fryer to 380ºF (193ºC).
2. Using a fork, poke 2 to 3 holes in the potatoes, then coat each with about ½ tablespoon olive oil and ½ teaspoon salt.
3. Place the potatoes into the air fryer basket and bake for 30 minutes.
4. Remove the potatoes from the air fryer, and slice in half. Using a spoon, scoop out the flesh of the potatoes, leaving a ½-inch layer of potato inside the skins, and set the skins aside.
5. In a medium bowl, combine the scooped potato middles with the remaining 2 tablespoons of olive oil, ½ teaspoon of salt, black pepper, and cilantro. Mix until well combined.
6. Divide the potato filling into the now-empty potato skins, spreading it evenly over them. Top each potato with a tablespoon each of the olives and feta.
7. Place the loaded potato skins back into the air fryer and bake for 15 minutes.
8. Serve with additional chopped cilantro or parsley and a drizzle of olive oil, if desired.

Per Serving
calories: 270 | fat: 13g | protein: 5g
carbs: 34g | fiber: 3g | sodium: 748mg

Tuna and Caper Croquettes

Prep time: 10 minutes | Cook time: 25 minutes | Makes 36 croquettes

6 tablespoons extra-virgin olive oil, plus 1 to 2 cups
5 tablespoons almond flour, plus 1 cup, divided
1¼ cups heavy cream
1 (4-ounce / 113-g) can olive oil-packed yellowfin tuna
1 tablespoon chopped red onion
2 teaspoons minced capers
½ teaspoon dried dill
¼ teaspoon freshly ground black pepper
2 large eggs
1 cup panko bread crumbs (or a gluten-free version)

1. In a large skillet, heat 6 tablespoons olive oil over medium-low heat. Add 5 tablespoons almond flour and cook, stirring constantly, until a smooth paste forms and the flour browns slightly, 2 to 3 minutes.
2. Increase the heat to medium-high and gradually add the heavy cream, whisking constantly until completely smooth and thickened, another 4 to 5 minutes.
3. Remove from the heat and stir in the tuna, red onion, capers, dill, and pepper.
4. Transfer the mixture to an 8-inch square baking dish that is well coated with olive oil and allow to cool to room temperature. Cover and refrigerate until chilled, at least 4 hours or up to overnight.
5. To form the croquettes, set out three bowls. In one, beat together the eggs. In another, add the remaining almond flour. In the third, add the panko. Line a baking sheet with parchment paper.
6. Using a spoon, place about a tablespoon of cold prepared dough into the flour mixture and roll to coat. Shake off excess and, using your hands, roll into an oval.
7. Dip the croquette into the beaten egg, then lightly coat in panko. Set on lined baking sheet and repeat with the remaining dough.
8. In a small saucepan, heat the remaining 1 to 2 cups of olive oil, so that the oil is about 1 inch deep, over medium-high heat. The smaller the pan, the less oil you will need, but you will need more for each batch.
9. Test if the oil is ready by throwing a pinch of panko into pot. If it sizzles, the oil is ready for frying. If it sinks, it's not quite ready. Once the oil is heated, fry the croquettes 3 or 4 at a time, depending on the size of your pan, removing with a slotted spoon when golden brown. You will need to adjust the temperature of the oil occasionally to prevent burning. If the croquettes get dark brown very quickly, lower the temperature.

Per Serving (3 croquettes)
calories: 245 | fat: 22g | protein: 6g
carbs: 7g | fiber: 1g | sodium: 85mg

Creamy Hummus

Prep time: 5 minutes | Cook time: 0 minutes | Serves 8

1 (15-ounce / 425-g) can garbanzo beans, rinsed and drained
2 cloves garlic, peeled
¼ cup lemon juice
1 teaspoon salt
¼ cup plain Greek yogurt
½ cup tahini paste
2 tablespoons extra-virgin olive oil, divided

1. Add the garbanzo beans, garlic cloves, lemon juice, and salt to a food processor fitted with a chopping blade. Blend for 1 minute, until smooth.
2. Scrape down the sides of the processor. Add the Greek yogurt, tahini paste, and 1 tablespoon of olive oil and blend for another minute, until creamy and well combined.
3. Spoon the hummus into a serving bowl. Drizzle the remaining tablespoon of olive oil on top.

Per Serving
calories: 189 | fat: 13g | protein: 7g
carbs: 14g | fiber: 4g | sodium: 313mg

Appendix 1: 4-Week Meal Plan

Week 1

DAYS	BREAKFAST	LUNCH	DINNER	SNACK/ DESSERT	REMINDER
1	Orange French Toast [19]	Couscous Confetti Salad[103]	Thyme Whole Roasted Red Snapper[34]	Whole Wheat Pita Chips[164]	Moderate Exercise; A Glass of Wine.
2	Cheesy Mini Frittatas[20]	Roasted Acorn Squash with Sage[72]	Beef and Potatoes with Tahini Sauce[64]	Grilled Fruit Skewers[140]	Moderate Exercise; A Glass of Wine.
3	Avocado Toast with Poached Eggs[22]	Rosemary Roasted Red Potatoes[72]	Greek Lemon Chicken Kebabs[53]	Greek-Style Potato Skins[164]	Moderate Exercise; A Glass of Wine.
4	Tomato, Herb, and Goat Cheese Frittata[24]	Baked Sweet Potato Black Bean Burgers[92]	Almond-Crusted Swordfish[40]	Creamy Hummus [165]	Moderate Exercise; A Glass of Wine.
5	Chickpea and Hummus Patties in Pitas[30]	Beet Summer Salad[126]	Dinner Meaty Baked Penne[117]	Crunchy Chili Chickpeas[153]	Moderate Exercise; A Glass of Wine.
6	Morning Creamy Iced Coffee[20]	Moroccan Chicken Meatballs[60]	Paella Soup[132]	Healthy Deviled Eggs with Greek Yogurt[154]	Moderate Exercise; A Glass of Wine.
7	Tuna and Avocado Salad Sandwich[26]	Tomato and Lentil Salad with Feta[119]	Linguine with Artichokes and Peas[114]	Baked Pears with Mascarpone Cheese[143]	Moderate Exercise; A Glass of Wine.

Week 2

DAYS	BREAKFAST	LUNCH	DINNER	SNACK/ DESSERT	REMINDER
1	Hearty Honey-Apricot Granola[28]	Grilled Lemon Shrimp[32]	Spatchcock Chicken with Lemon and Rosemary[52]	Fig Crostini with Mascarpone [138]	Moderate Exercise; A Glass of Wine.
2	Shakshuka with Cilantro[23]	Herb Lentil-Rice Balls[93]	Garlic Shrimp Black Bean Pasta[39]	Beet Chips [154]	Moderate Exercise; A Glass of Wine.
3	Pumpkin Muffins[24]	Bulgur Pilaf with Garbanzos[103]	Sea Bass Crusted with Moroccan Spices[41]	Spiced Cashews[154]	Moderate Exercise; A Glass of Wine.
4	Parmesan Spinach Pie[29]	Carrot and Bean Stuffed Peppers[72]	Rigatoni with Pancetta and Veggie[114]	Sweet Potato Chips[155]	Moderate Exercise; A Glass of Wine.
5	Fruity Pancakes with Berry-Honey Compote[26]	Italian Fried Shrimp[32]	Pork Tenderloin with Dijon Apple Sauce[68]	Cranberry Chocolate Granola Bars[155]	Moderate Exercise; A Glass of Wine.
6	Sweet Potato Toast[19]	Cod Saffron Rice[32]	Triple-Green Pasta with Parmesan[116]	Carrot Cake Cupcakes with Walnuts[155]	Moderate Exercise; A Glass of Wine.
7	Feta and Pepper Frittata[22]	Quinoa and Garbanzo Salad[119]	Classic Escabeche[36]	Spiced Roasted Chickpeas[156]	Moderate Exercise; A Glass of Wine.

Week 3

DAYS	BREAKFAST	LUNCH	DINNER	SNACK/ DESSERT	REMINDER
1	Mediterranean Herb Frittata[28]	Ratatouille [73]	Bean Balls with Marinara [95]	Blueberry, Pecan, and Oat Crisp[146]	Moderate Exercise; A Glass of Wine.
2	Healthy Green Smoothie [23]	Poached Chicken Breast with Romesco Sauce[51]	Olive Oil-Poached Tuna[42]	Homemade Trail Mix[156]	Moderate Exercise; A Glass of Wine.
3	Warm Bulgur Breakfast Bowls with Fruits[27]	Fast Seafood Paella[37]	Mushroom Parmesan Risotto[104]	Apple Chips with Chocolate Tahini Sauce[160]	Moderate Exercise; A Glass of Wine.
4	Pumpkin Layers with Honey Granola[20]	White Bean Soup with Kale[129]	Orzo with Shrimp and Feta Cheese [115]	Savory Mediterranean Spiced Popcorn [160]	Moderate Exercise; A Glass of Wine.
5	Polenta with Arugula, Figs, and Blue Cheese[29]	Avocado and Hearts of Palm Salad[120]	Brown Rice Bowls with Roasted Vegetables [109]	Citrus-Thyme Chickpeas [157]	Moderate Exercise; A Glass of Wine.
6	Blueberry and Chia Seeds Smoothie [21]	Roasted Asparagus and Tomatoes [74]	Chicken Thigh with Roasted Artichokes [55]	Crispy Seedy Crackers [157]	Moderate Exercise; A Glass of Wine.
7	Baked Ricotta with Honey Pears[25]	White Bean Lettuce Wraps[94]	Fideos with Seafood[34]	Nut Butter Cup[147]	Moderate Exercise; A Glass of Wine.

Week 4

DAYS	BREAKFAST	LUNCH	DINNER	SNACK/ DESSERT	REMINDER
1	Tangy Almond-Pistachio Smoothie **[27]**	Lentil Bulgur Pilaf**[104]**	Chicken Piccata with Mushrooms and Parsley **[56]**	Summer Strawberry Panna Cotta**[144]**	Moderate Exercise; A Glass of Wine.
2	Breakfast Pancakes with Berry Sauce**[26]**	Crispy Fried Sardines **[34]**	Asparagus and Grape Tomato Pasta**[116]**	Mediterranean-Style Trail Mix**[160]**	Moderate Exercise; A Glass of Wine.
3	Apple-Tahini Toast**[25]**	Vegetable Hummus Wraps**[76]**	Salmon with Tomatoes and Olives**[43]**	Orange Mug Cake**[143]**	Moderate Exercise; A Glass of Wine.
4	Banana Corn Fritters**[21]**	White Cannellini Bean Stew**[94]**	Peach-Glazed Chicken Drumsticks **[57]**	Turkish Spiced Mixed-Nuts**[159]**	Moderate Exercise; A Glass of Wine.
5	Feta and Olive Scrambled Eggs**[25]**	Turkish-Inspired Pinto Bean Salad**[94]**	Tilapia Fillet with Onion and Avocado**[45]**	Mediterranean Nutty Fat Bombs**[157]**	Moderate Exercise; A Glass of Wine.
6	Sweet Potato Toast**[19]**	Mushroom Barley Pilaf **[108]**	Sea Scallops with White Bean Purée**[40]**	Manchego Cheese Crackers**[163]**	Moderate Exercise; A Glass of Wine.
7	Veggie Stuffed Hash Browns**[23]**	Pasta Bean Soup**[135]**	Beef Short Ribs with Red Wine**[68]**	Lemony Peanut Butter Hummus**[164]**	Moderate Exercise; A Glass of Wine.

Appendix 2: Measurement Conversion Chart

VOLUME EQUIVALENTS(DRY)

US STANDARD	METRIC (APPROXIMATE)
1/8 teaspoon	0.5 mL
1/4 teaspoon	1 mL
1/2 teaspoon	2 mL
3/4 teaspoon	4 mL
1 teaspoon	5 mL
1 tablespoon	15 mL
1/4 cup	59 mL
1/2 cup	118 mL
3/4 cup	177 mL
1 cup	235 mL
2 cups	475 mL
3 cups	700 mL
4 cups	1 L

VOLUME EQUIVALENTS(LIQUID)

US STANDARD	US STANDARD (OUNCES)	METRIC (APPROXIMATE)
2 tablespoons	1 fl.oz.	30 mL
1/4 cup	2 fl.oz.	60 mL
1/2 cup	4 fl.oz.	120 mL
1 cup	8 fl.oz.	240 mL
1 1/2 cup	12 fl.oz.	355 mL
2 cups or 1 pint	16 fl.oz.	475 mL
4 cups or 1 quart	32 fl.oz.	1 L
1 gallon	128 fl.oz.	4 L

TEMPERATURES EQUIVALENTS

FAHRENHEIT(F)	CELSIUS(C) (APPROXIMATE)
225 °F	107 °C
250 °F	120 °C
275 °F	135 °C
300 °F	150 °C
325 °F	160 °C
350 °F	180 °C
375 °F	190 °C
400 °F	205 °C
425 °F	220 °C
450 °F	235 °C
475 °F	245 °C
500 °F	260 °C

WEIGHT EQUIVALENTS

US STANDARD	METRIC (APPROXIMATE)
1 ounce	28 g
2 ounces	57 g
5 ounces	142 g
10 ounces	284 g
15 ounces	425 g
16 ounces (1 pound)	455 g
1.5 pounds	680 g
2 pounds	907 g

Appendix 3: The Dirty Dozen and Clean Fifteen

The Environmental Working Group (EWG) is a nonprofit, nonpartisan organization dedicated to protecting human health and the environment Its mission is to empower people to live healthier lives in a healthier environment. This organization publishes an annual list of the twelve kinds of produce, in sequence, that have the highest amount of pesticide residue-the Dirty Dozen-as well as a list of the fifteen kinds ofproduce that have the least amount of pesticide residue-the Clean Fifteen.

THE DIRTY DOZEN

- The 2016 Dirty Dozen includes the following produce. These are considered among the year's most important produce to buy organic:

Strawberries	Spinach
Apples	Tomatoes
Nectarines	Bell peppers
Peaches	Cherry tomatoes
Celery	Cucumbers
Grapes	Kale/collard greens
Cherries	Hot peppers

- *The Dirty Dozen list contains two additional itemskale/collard greens and hot peppers-because they tend to contain trace levels of highly hazardous pesticides.*

THE CLEAN FIFTEEN

- The least critical to buy organically are the Clean Fifteen list. The following are on the 2016 list:

Avocados	Papayas
Corn	Kiw
Pineapples	Eggplant
Cabbage	Honeydew
Sweet peas	Grapefruit
Onions	Cantaloupe
Asparagus	Cauliflower
Mangos	

- *Some of the sweet corn sold in the United States are made from genetically engineered (GE) seedstock. Buy organic varieties of these crops to avoid GE produce.*

Appendix 4: Recipe Index